LIVING THE
LIFE
UNEXPECTED

LIVING THE
LIFE
UNEXPECTED

12 WEEKS TO
YOUR PLAN B FOR
A MEANINGFUL AND
FULFILLING FUTURE
WITHOUT
CHILDREN

JODY DAY

bluebird
books for life

First self-published as *Rocking the Life Unexpected* in 2013

This revised and updated edition published in the UK 2016 by Bluebird
an imprint of Pan Macmillan
20 New Wharf Road, London N1 9RR
Associated companies throughout the world
www.panmacmillan.com

ISBN 978-1-5098-0903-5

1 3 5 7 9 8 6 4 2

A CIP catalogue record for this book is available from the British Library.

Typeset by Richard Marston, www.richardmarston.com
Printed and bound by CPI Group (UK) Ltd, Croydon, CR0 4YY

Visit **www.panmacmillan.com** to read more about all our books
and to buy them. You will also find features, author interviews and
news of any author events, and you can sign up for e-newsletters
so that you're always first to hear about our new releases.

For Elly and Mark

Contents

Introduction

This book is written by a woman who wanted to be a mother and it didn't work out. And that, as you know, is a whole book in itself!

You'll be pleased to know that this book isn't going to tell you to 'get over it', point out that your childlessness isn't actually 'that big a deal', remind you 'how lucky you are that you don't have children', or even suggest that you explore adoption as your obvious next step. Because the fact is, we've all heard variations on these themes far too often. Whilst mothers and others rarely *mean* to hurt our feelings or insult our intelligence, it's often how we end up feeling ...

This book is about what I learned as I pulled myself out from the despair and heartbreak of my childlessness, and how I found a way to make my life feel meaningful again. It's about the network I created, Gateway Women, and the programme I developed so that I could share my experience of recovery from childlessness with other women, and guide them as they took the steps towards their own Plan B. An earlier version of this book was self-published in 2013, made possible by the crowd-funded support of Gateway Women from around the world, to whom I will always be incredibly grateful. This new, completely revised and expanded edition also includes the thoughts and experiences of some of the childless women (and men) I've had the privilege to get to know over the last few years. Their voices add that sense of being part of a tribe and I'd like to say a heartfelt thank you to each of them for sharing their private thoughts and feelings with me and with you.

I remember a particularly low moment in my life when I was feeling deeply unhappy and lost. I was forty-two and considering whether to take a job working with a voluntary organisation in Kabul, but decided against it in the end because I'd have to start my contract in October and I couldn't face the idea of how cold I'd be in the Afghan winter. You see, I wasn't bothered about getting shot or blown up, but I couldn't cope with the idea of getting cold! Looking back on this now, it's clear to me that I felt my life as a childless woman was so worthless that I didn't think that losing it would be such a big deal. After all, it's not like my kids and husband needed me, did they? My by-then ex-husband was lost deep in the throes of addiction, and I was beginning to realise that it was increasingly unlikely that I was ever going to become a mother.

Today I love my life again, and being able to guide and support other women as they learn to love *theirs* once more brings me great joy and satisfaction. If I had my time over, I'd still wish to be a mother, but these days I'm genuinely fine with the way things have turned out. Really, I'm not faking it! I find I'm able to enjoy the advantages of *not* being a mother, take pleasure in being around other people's children and enjoy planning my future. I call that having a Plan B and this book is going to help you start moving towards yours.

Together, we're going to begin creating your Plan B for a meaningful and fulfilling future without children.

Here's to new beginnings.

How to Use This Book

This book is going to introduce you to some new ways to think and feel about your situation as a childless woman. It's based very closely on the workshops and courses that I've been running since 2011, although I've selected and adapted the exercises to make them a little easier for you to do on your own or as part of your own self-organised reading group.

Because of the new thoughts and feelings that this work brings up, I recommend that you read just one chapter each week and then take a break to do the exercises and see what comes up for you. This will give you time to reflect on what you've learned, unlearned and discovered, and to begin to integrate that into your new awareness. You might also want to keep a journal throughout this process, as it can be very helpful. However, if you prefer to read the book through from beginning to end and do the exercises as you go, or afterwards, that will serve you well too. You might be one of those people who *mean* to do the exercises in books but rarely do (guilty as charged!). You'll be missing some of the richness, but do whatever works for you. After all, you're probably fed up with obeying other people's rules anyway . . .

This book can also be used as a framework for holding your own twelve-session reading group with other childless women, either in person or online. The exercises can be done in a group setting and this can be really powerful – either by allowing you to see how similar your responses are (when you believed you were the only woman who had those thoughts) or to hear and be exposed to new ways of thinking that hadn't occurred to you. Each chapter ends with 'Reflections', which can act as a helpful conversational starting point for the beginning of each group session. If you'd like more information on how to host and run a live or online reading group, you'll find more information on the Gateway Women website.

One thing I would *really* recommend you do right now is the 'Plan B Healing Inventory' questionnaire, which you'll find on the next page. You can also print out a copy of this from the Gateway Women website. This will preserve a snapshot of your thoughts and feelings about your situation today and can be a valuable way of tracking how things have changed for you once you get to the end of the book. However, like everything else written here, I'd like to stress that this is an *invitation*, not an instruction. Part of recovery from childlessness is learning to trust yourself again, so I trust that you'll do what's right for you.

Plan B Healing Inventory

Please score the following questions on a scale of 0 to 10, once before you read the book and then again afterwards. You can also come back to this questionnaire annually as it can be a really helpful way to see how you're progressing, and where you might need to focus to get to an even better place.

		Date:	Date:
		0–10	0–10
1	How easy do you find it being around your friends and family's children? (From 0, *'I do all I can to avoid it, it's so hard'* to 10, *'Absolutely fine, no problem at all'*)		
2	How easy do you find it to talk to people about your situation and history? (From 0, *'I'd rather the floor opened up and swallowed me'* to 10, *'No problem'*)		
3	How hard do you find it when people ask you if you have kids? (From 0, *'I want to run away rather than answer it'* to 10, *'Pretty dull question but not painful'*)		
4	How comfortable are you holding a baby in your arms? (From 0, *'I simply won't do it'* to 10, *'It's a delightful experience!'*)		

5 How much do you believe that there are other ways to experience the joy, connection and meaning in life that mothers seem to have?
(From 0, *'I simply don't believe it's possible'* to 10, *'It's absolutely possible'*)

6 How angry are you about how things have turned out?
(From 0, *'So angry I could self-combust'* to 10, *'I'm at peace with how things turned out these days'*)

7 How much do you blame other people for how things have turned out?
(From 0, *'Others are totally to blame'* to 10, *'I've worked through it now'*)

8 How sad are you about how things have turned out?
(From 0, *'I'm totally heartbroken'* to 10, *'I rarely feel sad about how things have turned out anymore'*)

9 How much do you enjoy the benefits that come with not having children?
(From 0, *'What benefits?'* to 10, *'I enjoy them to the max!'*)

10 How bothered are you with how people may perceive you as a childless woman?
(From 0, *'I utterly hate the way people see me!'* to 10, *'I don't let it bother me any more'*)

11 How aware are you of inspiring childless women role models?
(From 0, *'There aren't any'* to 10, *'I'm aware and excited there are so many!'*)

12 How strong is your mojo these days?
(From 0, *'Dead and buried'* to 10, *'On fire!'*)

13 How full of clutter is your home?
(From 0, *'I haven't seen the floor in a long time'* to
10, *'It's pretty organised actually'*)

14 How are you keeping up with finances and other
'life admin' tasks these days?
(From 0, *'My paperwork and finances are a train
wreck'* to 10, *'I'm totally on top of it all'*)

15 How comfortable are you with the idea of taking
risks and doing things differently?
(From 0, *'Absolutely no way'*, to 10, *'Totally up for
it!'*)

16 How often do you really laugh your head off these
days?
(From 0, *'I don't remember the last time I laughed'*,
to 10, *'I love how much I laugh now!'*)

17 How willing are you to let go of the dream of
motherhood?
(From 0, *'No way!'* to 10, *'I've let it go'*)

18 How often do you pleasantly daydream about your
childless future?
(From 0, *'How is that even possible?'* to 10, *'A lot –
there's a lot to look forward to again!'*)

19 How often do you worry about your childless
future?
(From 0, *'I worry myself sick'* to 10, *'I'm involved in
planning it rather than worrying about it'*)

20 How well do you take care of your body?
(From 0, *'What body?'* to 10, *'Physically, I've never taken better care of myself than now'*)

21 How happy are you with the way you look?
(From 0, *'I wouldn't know, I don't look'* to 10, *'I'm looking the best I've done in years!'*)

22 How connected to your inner world do you feel?
(From 0, *'I avoid it'* to 10, *'I'm feeling really in touch with it'*)

23 How kind are you to yourself?
(From 0, *'Why the hell would I be "kind" to myself?'* to 10, *'As kind as possible'*)

24 How nurturing and 'mothering' is your inner dialogue?
(From 0, *'Not at all!'* to 10, *'I'm my own best friend – nurturing, kind and supportive'*)

25 How much do you enjoy your work?
(From 0, *'I absolutely loathe it'* to 10, *'I love my work and find it very fulfilling'*)

26 How much do you feel like an outsider in your workplace or with colleagues?
(From 0, *'I'm the office freak'* to 10, *'I feel accepted for who I am and I'm comfortable with my difference'*)

27 How creative do you think you are?
(From 0, *'Not a creative cell in my body'* to 10, *'Creativity is a vital part of my life'*)

28 How much play is there in your daily life?
(From 0, *'A slug is more playful than me'* to 10, *'I find play pretty well much everywhere!'*)

29 How many minor illnesses do you get?
(From 0, *'I'm sure to catch anything going round'* to 10, *'I get sick very rarely'*)

30 How much do you believe that you're capable of finding a Plan B?
(From 0, *'I don't believe it at all'* to 10, *'I feel totally confident that I can do this'*)

31 How much of you is scared that you're uniquely equipped to fail at life?
(From 0, *'Failure is my middle name'* to 10, *'I'm not a failure; I can do this!'*)

32 How important is meaning to you?
(From 0, *'Meaning is only for mothers'* to 10, *'Creating and sustaining meaning in my life is absolutely vital for me'*)

33 How much do you worry about growing old without children?
(From 0, *'I'm absolutely terrified'* to 10, *'I've made all my plans and I'm hoping it's going to be pretty good!'*)

34 How much importance do you give to leaving a legacy?
(From 0, *'What kind of legacy could I possibly leave?'* to 10, *'It's really important to me and something I'm actively working on'*)

35	How much do you believe that you personally are capable of making a contribution to this world other than by being a mother? (From 0, *'Are you joking?'* to 10, *'Not only am I capable of doing so, but I am doing it'*)		
36	How connected, stimulated and supported do you feel by your current social circle? (From 0, *'What social circle? I live under a rock'* to 10, *'My friendship group is vibrant, varied and supportive and growing all the time'*)		
37	How much time do you spend with other childless women who are working towards (or who are already living) their Plan B? (From 0, *'None, there aren't any, and certainly not round here'* to 10, *'I couldn't imagine my life without the great group of childless friends I've made!'*)		
38	How far along in your recovery from childlessness do you think you are? (From 0, *'Rock bottom'* to 10, *'I feel that I've done the work to integrate this loss into who I've become (and am becoming!) and feel strong and whole again'*)		
39	How happy are you to be alive? (From 0, *'I'm existing, that's all'* to 10, *'I'm thrilled and delighted to be alive!'*)		
40	How ready are you to live the life unexpected? (From 0, *'Not at all, never was and doubt I ever will be'* to 10, *'Bring it on!'*)		
	Total		

An Overview of This Book's Structure

Although this book has a linear twelve-chapter structure, within that structure is an ebb and flow between the deeply personal and the more public, societal aspects of being a childless woman today. In working with childless women in groups and workshops, I have found that this structure helps to gently reveal layers of stuck thought and feeling and enables a gradual progression of 'aha' moments that work together in an integrated way.

For some of us, placing our own experience within a broader context helps us to realise that we really aren't the *only* women that this has happened to, which can be a huge relief, and may signal the start of us challenging our shame-based internal monologues. However, for others, this might feel too heady and intellectual and they'd rather dive straight into working with their individual felt experience and come back to some of the societal stuff later.

Because of this structure, you may find that some parts of this book feel more relevant to you right now. So, in order for you to assess this, here is a brief overview of each chapter.

- **Chapter 1: The Power of Our Stories**
  The book starts at a very personal level with my story and looks at the power of our stories in shaping our lives. It explores some of the many different experiences that may have led to us being childless, other than the simplistic dichotomy of 'didn't want' or 'couldn't have', and includes the stories of other women from around the world in their own words.

- **Chapter 2: You're Not Alone**
  We now pull back to survey the broader social and economic context that has led to almost one in five women (20 per cent) of our generation reaching the age of forty-five without having had children, as opposed to the historical rate of one in ten (10 per cent). We

take a look at childlessness around the world as well as what the French and Swedish governments do differently to other countries to achieve the lowest rates of childlessness in the developed world.

- **Chapter 3: Motherhood with a Capital 'M'**
  In this chapter we explore how and why motherhood has become such a minefield of social expectations and pressures for women (both those with and without children). We also begin to examine our own childhood experiences and what messages we may have picked up that have influenced our beliefs and choices concerning motherhood and childlessness.

- **Chapter 4: Working Through the Grief of Childlessness**
  Grief over childlessness is an issue for us at personal, social and cultural levels, so in this chapter we take a new look at what grief is (and surprisingly, why it's a good thing). We explore how grief impacts us personally (whether grieving as a couple or solo), and what we can do to process it so that we are ready to embrace our lives again.

- **Chapter 5: Liberating Yourself from the Opinion of Others**
  This chapter examines the cultural landscape of how, as childless women, we can be pigeonholed into a few reductive and mostly rather unkind stereotypes. We explore why that might be, whether within our family of origin, at work or even at the hairdresser, and what we can do to reframe our experiences, choose our own labels and celebrate our own role models.

- **Chapter 6: Who Moved My Mojo?**
  For childless women, the loss of the potential identity of mother can be devastating to our ego and sense of who we are – and thus demolish our mojo, our joie de vivre. This chapter provides an insight into why this might be, and how putting meaning back at the centre of our new lives is an important step in getting our mojo back.

- **Chapter 7: Letting Go of Your Burned-out Dreams**

  Letting go of the dream of motherhood is, for most of us, a very painful experience. In this chapter, we explore what happens when either most of our life force was channelled into this dream, or, conversely, how unexplored ambivalence held us back. Acknowledging the need to understand, grieve and let go of our unfulfilled dreams is vital in order for new dreams to arise.

- **Chapter 8: Reconnecting to Your Source**

  This chapter looks at how our relationship with our body has been affected by our childlessness, and how for many of us this may have led to a cycle of punishing or disconnecting from it as a way to avoid emotional pain. We explore how healing our relationship with our body can be a powerful route to healing our relationship with life, and ultimately with joy.

- **Chapter 9: The Mother Within**

  We now begin to unpack the relationship we have with ourselves in our head and heart, and look at the source of some of our shaming and hyper-critical internal monologues. We learn how becoming a 'good enough mother' to ourselves can be a compassionate and effective way to transform our inner world.

- **Chapter 10: Creating a Life for Yourself as a Childless Woman**

  The idea of being creative seems to strike fear into the heart of many of us, often because we have a very narrow idea of what creativity means. However, without an element of play in our lives, we can feel deadened. Creativity, play and change are important. I can feel your fear already ... (Please don't skip this chapter!)

- **Chapter 11: Putting Your Plan B Together**

  Plan B isn't a new job, a new city or a new relationship. It's a fundamental refurbishment of your life from the inside out. In this chapter we debunk some of the common myths about Plan Bs and introduce you to the forensic tools you'll use to start exploring what *your* Plan B needs to include to create a meaningful and fulfilling future without children.

- **Chapter 12: Taking Off the Invisibility Cloak**
  It's time to celebrate, collaborate and agitate! In this final chapter we look at ways in which we can come together as childless women and end our isolation by reaching out and staying connected to each other. We also consider what our wider social influence might be as powerful, connected, liberated, aware, intelligent, independent older women. We contemplate what our legacy might be if it's not the children or grandchildren we expected to have, and also take a good, hard look at our fears about ageing without children.

- **Appendix**
  As these resources are constantly evolving, you can find a fuller, more up-to-date version of them on the Gateway Women website at www.gateway-women.com.
  Resources – organisations, blogs, websites, forums and other resources from around the world for childless women.
  Recommended Reading – books that I've read and which have supported me, and others, as we heal from our childlessness and move towards our Plan B.

- **Acknowledgements**
  A thank you to all of you who have helped make this book possible.

- **Endnotes**
  References from the text of this book. Also available online at bit.ly/LTLU-Bluebird.

A Note on Terminology

In this book, I define 'childless' as being without a biological child of your own when you had hoped you would have one someday, whether that's because of infertility or for any of the many other ways that it might not have happened. 'Childless' can be a bit of a harsh word, but I don't need to tell *you* how harsh it feels sometimes.

I really like the word 'childfree', but this term (or its abbreviation 'CF' or 'CBC' – childfree-by-choice) refers to those women (and men) who have actively *chosen* not to have children. Many of them have insisted since childhood that they didn't want children and have never changed their mind, even though they were often told that they would, 'one day'.

'Childless-by-circumstance' rather than 'childless-by-choice' seems to be the term that describes our situation unambiguously, even though I'm aware that those 'circumstances' can often be fraught with ambiguity!

There are many other terms in use, including the acronym 'nomo' (not-mother), which I created and which I explore in more depth later. But for now, as you read on, in its simplest terms:

- childless = circumstantial (including infertility)
- childfree = chosen
- nomo = not-mother (for whatever reason, by choice or not)

About Me: Jody Day

I set up the Gateway Women friendship and support network in 2011 with the aim of supporting, inspiring and empowering childless women like myself to develop meaningful and fulfilling lives without children. It's grown hugely and I now run groups, workshops, social events and retreats both on and offline, as well as giving regular public talks. We have Meetup groups in towns and cities across the world: in the UK and Ireland, Europe, USA, Canada, Australia, New Zealand and South Africa. There's also a private Gateway Women online community with members from all over the English-speaking world. Finally, we have our own 'school gates' network!

My own experience of coming to terms with my childlessness was hard, lonely and scary, and I wanted to make it easier for other women to make this transition. And I wanted some company too, in this new and unexpected part of my life as a childless woman, because the loneliness and isolation of being a nomo in a culture that seems to have gone motherhood-crazy took me completely by surprise.

As Gateway Women has grown and become more influential, I'm regularly asked to speak in public and am often interviewed in the press. Sometimes I feel like the 'taboo girl' as I've become so comfortable talking about the things that our society still regards as shameful, such as medical infertility, social infertility (not having a suitable partner during our potentially fertile years), being single, menopause, grief and ageing without children. My Plan B turns out to be becoming a voice for childless women and I love it! Increasingly I'm talking with healthcare providers, academics and social policy-makers as I'm determined to get our needs and our presence acknowledged, understood and onto the public agenda.

There's a lot to do to educate people about the stigmas and prejudices we face at present from our friends, families, colleagues, employers, medical professionals, governments and the media. We are one in five women turning forty-five, with perhaps an even greater proportion coming up behind us; the time has come for our voice to be heard and our influence to be felt. We have so much to offer to the world, but first we need to believe that ourselves ...

It's my mission to get the message out there that it's not only possible to *survive* involuntary childlessness, but to *thrive* as a childless woman, and to create a meaningful and fulfilling life without children. I really hope that this book and the support of other like-minded childless women helps you to let go of some of your sadness and move towards your future with a spring in your step again.

Together, we can do this, and more. But first, you have to heal. And for that, you need your sisters. You've found them.

Welcome to your tribe.

The room called
CHILDLESSNESS
has many doors;
not just ones marked
'DIDN'T WANT'
or
'COULDN'T
HAVE'.

CHAPTER 1

The Power of Our Stories

If you hoped, planned and expected to become a mother one day, but it didn't work out, this book is for you.

Wow! What a universe of pain, heartbreak, surprise, dashed hopes, shock and grief are contained in that one short sentence. Pain that the rest of society, our family, colleagues, close friends and often even our partners may find difficult to understand. Or if they do, their help may come in the form of well-meaning but painful comments or advice that can often end up making us feel worse. So we learn that perhaps keeping quiet about our feelings is the safest option . . .

Almost one in five women in the UK and USA have reached their mid-forties without having had children: some of them by choice, many of them by circumstance. In other developed countries, such as Italy, it's one in four, and as high as one in three for Japan and Germany.*

Although most people who don't know our story may imagine that we either chose not to have children or couldn't have them, the truth of our experiences is far more complex. And indeed, recent research meta-analysis suggests that whilst perhaps 10 per cent of women without children choose not to be mothers (childfree), and 10 per cent

* See Chapter 2 for a more detailed analysis of this data.

couldn't have them for medical reasons including infertility, 80 per cent of childless women are 'childless by circumstance'.¹ To explore the range of ways that we can be childless, I've pulled together some of the many ways it can happen, but by no means is it an exhaustive list. As you read through it, you might like to keep a note of the number of any factor that applies to your story. It might end up looking like an order for a Chinese takeaway, but bear with me!

Fifty Ways Not to Be a Mother

1. Being single and not finding a suitable relationship to bring children into.

2. Being unknowingly misinformed about our fertility and not realising that after thirty-five it's half what it was at twenty-five, and that by the time we're forty we have only a very small number of viable eggs left. The age that many women think they need to worry about is forty, when in fact it's much younger.

3. Not meeting a partner until we're past our childbearing years.

4. Realising that because of our sexuality, the journey was always going to involve IVF, and when we did try IVF, it didn't work.

5. Being unable to afford to bring up a child on our own as well as working to support them (and pay for childcare) so that we are therefore unable to 'go it alone' or be considered for adoption.

6. Being scared of having children because of our own difficult childhood before realising too late that we were not condemned to repeat this with our own children.

7. Being brought up mostly by our mothers following the relationship breakdown of our parents, and having seen the emotional, logistical and financial struggle of single parenthood, we were determined to find a 'stable' partnership before having children, but were unable to find one, or not in time.

8. Spending our thirties healing childhood wounds in therapy, and then finding it too late to find a healthy partner and start a family.

9. Recovering from addiction issues right at the end of our fertile years.

10. Having a partner with addiction or mental health issues that took up a great deal of time and energy until it was too late to have children.

11. Being in an emotionally and/or physically abusive relationship that destroyed our confidence so much that we left it too long to leave, recover and find a suitable partner with whom to have children.

12. Not making motherhood a priority and somehow expecting it to 'just happen' one day.

13. Waiting for our partner to come round to the idea of having a family, only to find out as we approach the end of our fertility that they've decided they definitely don't want children, or still 'not yet' …

14. Chronically painful periods as a teenager, dismissed as 'something you'll grow out of' when in fact it was endometriosis, which led to chronic pain, difficulty conceiving and carrying a baby to term and sometimes a hysterectomy.

15. Infertility issues of our own.

16. Infertility issues of our partner.

17. Infertility issues of both partners.

18. Failed infertility treatments.

19. Miscarriage and early-term loss.

20. Stillbirth, cot death, early infancy mortality.

21. Choosing to 'go it alone' as a solo mother with sperm and/or egg donation but, after multiple attempts, not being successful.

22. Being with a partner who has had a vasectomy and for whom the reversal doesn't work.

23. Being educated at an academically focused school that placed a huge emphasis on pursuing a career and gave the impression that motherhood was not something to think about or aim for.

24. Adopting a child and then finding that although everyone now thinks you're a mother, you still feel 'childless' and guilty about it.

25. Adopting a child (or children), only for the adoption to break down at some point, sometimes due to the birth parents wishing (and being allowed) to parent their children again or due to the unmanageable severity of the child's behavioural difficulties.

26. Being unable to adopt because of being single (without meeting the right criteria), having insufficient funds, being the wrong age, being the wrong gender or sexual orientation, being the wrong ethnicity, being disabled, having had cancer, being too fat, not having a garden, being estranged from your own family, etc.

27. Staying in a relationship that we don't feel comfortable bringing children into.

28. Being in an unconsummated or sexually inactive relationship.

29. Being widowed.

30. Being born without a fully developed reproductive system or with genetic issues, such as Turner's Syndrome, leading to insufficient or non-existent ovarian reserve.

31. Our own or our partner's changed sexual orientation leading to relationship breakdown.

32. Not feeling comfortable having IVF or other treatments, or having them explicitly frowned upon by our faith, family or other significant influencers.

33. Being unable to afford fertility treatments, or to afford to continue.

34. Being denied fertility treatments.

35. Our partner or ourselves being ill during our most fertile years and so waiting for one or both to regain health.

36. Caring for a sick, elderly, disabled or vulnerable family member or friend during our fertile years.

37. Being a 'young carer' and parenting our younger siblings in our mother's place (due to illness, absence, death, addiction, depression, etc.) and thus believing that we'd 'had enough of mothering', only to realise too late that we would have liked to have had children of our own.

38. Losing a key relationship because of family disapproval on religious, cultural, class, financial or other grounds, and then not meeting another partner in time to start a family.

39. Medical conditions that make becoming a parent difficult.

40. Having genetic inheritance issues of our own, or our partner's, that make us decide not to risk having children.

41. Needing to save enough money to buy a home and pay off student debts before we could afford to start a family, only for it to be too late.

42. Being with a partner who already has children and doesn't want more.

43. Being with a partner who doesn't want children at all (a childfree partner).

44. Becoming a stepmother and finding your partner's parenting style so off-putting we choose not to have children with them, or we'd like to but we feel it would be just too painful for our partner's children to cope with.

45. Being unable to get pregnant with the eggs we froze when we were younger.

46. Being ambivalent about motherhood and realising too late that we really *do* want a family.

47. Finding out that the man who said he wanted children was lying as he'd had a vasectomy and hadn't told us.

48. Finding donor egg treatment something we don't feel comfortable

pursuing, isn't legal in our country or we can't afford, thereby bringing our fertility treatments to an end.

49. Finding surrogacy as an alternative to having our own baby something we don't feel comfortable with, isn't legal in our country or we can't afford.

50. Having our ovaries damaged by chemotherapy and our partner being unwilling to consider egg donation.

I could keep going, but I think you get my point – behind every woman without children is a story, often many stories woven together into a complex pattern of pain and disappointment. Your story may be one of these, or a patchwork of them, or it may be number 51. I'm absolutely sure the list could go on for much longer ...

Most people think that we either chose not to have children or that we couldn't. The truth is far more complex ...

My Story

I got married young (although I thought I was very grown-up at the time) at twenty-six. My husband, seven years older than me, was a charming, glamorous fashion designer and we fell madly in love. I wasn't completely sure I wanted children when we married and I told my husband-to-be so; having had a pretty disrupted childhood myself, 'family life' wasn't my idea of fun.

But gradually I got used to the idea, and because it was no longer an abstract notion of 'children', but a child who would be the product of our love and made up of our combined DNA, when I was twenty-nine we started trying for a family. I had my own PR consultancy by then, but I gave it up to put my skills into helping my husband's new interior design business grow. After all, my thinking went, *his* was the business that was going to support us 'as a family'. Looking back on it now, I can't quite believe how little thought I gave to these decisions; it's like I was following a script and yet if you'd asked me at the time, I would have said that I was an independent thinker.

The interior design business thrived and we worked very well together, but I didn't get pregnant. I wasn't too concerned; I'd had an abortion at twenty, which, although it was pretty traumatic emotionally (I was terrified of having a baby as one of the messages I'd internalised from family, school and wider society was that 'children ruin your life') at least it reassured me that 'everything worked'. I was more confused than anything else at my inability to get pregnant because it didn't fit in with my plans – and I was a ferocious planner in those days! I cringe to admit it now but I had a chart listing month-by-month my plans for the next five years of my life, including which months I aimed to conceive so that our children's births would fit around our schedule. I still have that chart in a box somewhere; I keep it to remind me how much I've changed, and how I no longer expect life to go according to my plans.

At the age of thirty-three, and four years into trying for a baby, I had a laparoscopy under general anaesthetic – a procedure in which a camera is inserted through your navel to take a look around the reproductive system. 'Ready to move into!' said my avuncular gynaecologist as I came round from the anaesthetic. 'Excellent property! Nothing to worry about!' All the tests on hormones, sperm counts, etc., came back fine too. Looking back on it now, I can't quite believe that after trying to conceive for four years, IVF wasn't even mentioned to us by the doctors, nor was I given any advice about the fact that I only had two years before I turned thirty-five and statistically my fertility fell off a cliff. They reassured us that everything was fine, that there was no damage from the abortion, and I was happy to take that at face value.

Over the coming years, we kept on trying (the only advice we ever got from doctors) and I saw every nutritionist, herbalist, acupuncturist, shaman, healer, homoeopath, naturopath and quack in London. I tried every diet, made all the lifestyle changes and became an expert on my ovulation dates, peeing on every colour and type of stick I could buy. Yet, each month, regular as clockwork, my period would come and I'd be in tears once more.

The doctors called it 'unexplained infertility' and left it at that, never mentioning that we may have been eligible for one or two rounds of IVF treatment paid for by our local health authority. We did briefly consider IVF, but couldn't afford it privately and I was very wary of it too – I really didn't like the idea of the hormone treatments and I was convinced I'd conceive naturally anyway. I mean *absolutely, unshakably convinced*. All these years later, and with the benefit of hindsight, I can see that perhaps my earlier ambivalence over having a family may have found a new home – in my anti-IVF stance. And by the time I *was* ready to consider IVF, at thirty-seven, our marriage was not just on the rocks; it was most of the way up the beach. My husband's dashing personality had tipped over into chronic alcoholism and addiction and our lives had become hell. At thirty-eight, our marriage was over.

Astonishingly, I *still* thought there was plenty of time left for me to have a family! I reasoned that because I was young-looking for my age, that my periods were regular as clockwork and that I felt myself ovulating every month, it *must* have been my husband.

On a conscious level, I gave it no more thought and set my mind to getting divorced as quickly as possible and moving on. However, looking back, I can see that perhaps the subconscious pressure of babymania was pushing me to take fast, drastic action. I wonder now, had I not been so desperate for a child, if I would have stayed with my husband and fought for the marriage. But then again, fighting against addiction is never a fairly matched game, and I doubt I would have won. But as all childless women know, we always wonder how things would have turned out if . . .

Around the age of forty, I started dating again, and just before my forty-first birthday, my ex-husband got a casual girlfriend accidentally pregnant. She either didn't keep the baby or had a very early miscarriage – I can't remember now, the details are hazy with distress. But I do recall how the knowledge of this absolutely devastated me because I could no longer hold on to the fantasy that somehow things were going to work out 'naturally' for me.

In the next few years I had a couple of serious relationships, but sadly neither of them were stable enough to consider doing IVF. And so, when my most serious post-divorce relationship ended, I was forty-four years old. Well, forty-four and a half actually!

I remember a gloomy, rainy February afternoon in the grotty studio flat I'd moved into after a stormy and distressing break-up. I was standing watching the rain on the window when the traffic in the street seemed to become completely muted. In that moment, I became acutely aware of myself, standing there, looking out of the window. And then it came to me:

It's over. I'm never going to have a baby.

I realised with absolute clarity and complete certainty that even if I *were* to meet a new partner immediately, we'd need to be together for at least a year before we could even *think* about doing IVF. It was too late for that. I was too old.

It was over. I was never going to have a baby.

But instead of falling apart, something remarkable happened. I fell together.

These days, I feel comfortable calling it an epiphany. It started as a strong physical sensation in my belly that all the energy I'd been using to run each of the two separate 'versions' of my life all those years somehow merged back together. It was an odd feeling, as if the Jody who had been going to be a mother one day, and who'd been my constant shadow for the last fifteen years, reintegrated with the rest of me – the life I was actually living.

Then another new thought popped up: I thought back to when I'd been twenty, and how I used to survey the vast landscape of time ahead of me until I turned fifty and how I optimistically imagined that this gave me enough space to achieve whatever I set my sights on. My next new thought said: *If the years from twenty to fifty can feel like that, why can't the years from forty-five to seventy-five feel the same? As long as my health holds out, surely I can achieve something pretty significant in that time?*

I stood still, shocked: When was the last time I had thought something like that?!

Over the rest of the day, feelings and thoughts that I hadn't had for years started to bubble up. Amongst the wreckage of my life, I saw the beginnings of a new kind of hope. It was startling because I hadn't been able to imagine a future other than motherhood for such a long time that I'd forgotten that one could exist. It had been a baby or, well, nothing: a cliff of nothingness that I imagined falling off, leaving me hurtling downwards forever. The few times I *had* imagined alternative futures I'd learned to quash them, fearful that somehow even *thinking* about them would nix my chances of becoming a mother.

I'd love to say that, hallelujah, I was fixed from that moment forwards. But the truth is that what happened that day is that I came out of denial about my situation. I no longer saw my childlessness as a temporary situation on the way to motherhood, but as a permanent one. I was a childless woman, and would always be so. I am so grateful that I received a hint that day of what lay in my future, as I then entered a period of profound grief for the children I would never have, the life I would never live. But I had no idea it was grief – it would have been a huge help if I'd known ...

Soon after I was accepted onto a course to train as a psychotherapist and was due to start the following year. It was something I'd wanted to do for almost ten years but had kept putting aside. *Commit to a five-year course? What if I had a baby?* The training gave me an opportunity to start processing my sadness, introduced me to new ways to think about things and new friends to talk about them with.

About a year later, I started writing about being childless in a motherhood-mad world on a new blog I started: Gateway Women. I told it like it was and as I wrote about my situation and had the kind of frank, online discussions with women that I'd been longing to have for years, women from all over the world wrote back and said, 'Thank God I'm not the only one ...' or 'Thank you for finally telling the truth ...'

After a lot of encouragement, I gave my first public talk to a tiny audience of eight women, and was almost sick with anxiety. A journalist came and later interviewed me for a national newspaper and before long I was on the radio and in the media regularly. After each bit of publicity, I'd receive loads of emails from women asking for my help. So, with my heart in my mouth and feeling hugely nervous, I started the first Gateway Women group to see if I really could help others find their way through childlessness. Running that group was life-changing for me, and I've held it many times now, learning as much as I've taught thanks to the gutsy, pioneering women who've dared to break the taboo of talking about being childless. I also run weekend workshops and retreats, give regular public talks and am often in the media as I'm still one of the very few women who is prepared to be named and photographed and to talk openly about her childlessness.

Not having a family broke my heart. Some may think that's melodramatic, but I know it's true. However, grieving that loss and the life I longed for healed my heart, leaving it bigger than it was before.

The grief process changed me profoundly, and in ways I am still discovering. Several years on from that February afternoon I can say that although the sadness of not being a mother will always be a part of who I am, it no longer defines me.

You never 'get over' childlessness, but it is possible to heal around it. My childlessness was once an open wound and getting through each day was as much as I could do; I was the walking wounded. Now that wound has healed into a scar and I can live with a scar, dance with a scar, dream with a scar. It's a part of me now, though it will always be a tender spot. I loved my unborn children and they will always be with me, but now my life goes forward with them safely inside my heart forever.

Why Our Stories Matter

Throughout human history, stories have been the way that information has been remembered, honoured and passed on. Before we were able to record them in writing, storytelling was the only way that a community's history and culture could be handed down.

Who we are, and who we believe ourselves to be, is to a huge degree the result of the stories we tell ourselves.

We may think that our memory is accurate, but it is highly selective, like the editor of a news channel. If the data doesn't fit 'our story', we may choose not to notice it or, if we do notice it, to discount, diminish or forget it. Indeed, recent experiments in neuroscience have shown that 'the more often you remember something, the less accurate the memory becomes'.[2]

As childless women, our stories are currently invisible – our individual experience seems to exist in a cultural vacuum. In vain, we look for our reflection in films, books, on TV and in magazines, but we're not there. Or if we are, it's probably as a sad first-person confessional, a social commentary about the impending demographic disaster of an ageing population, or as a warning to younger women to get pregnant as soon as possible (if only it were that simple!). Women around the age of forty still hoping to have a family are routinely either pitied or ridiculed, whilst older childless women are disregarded or mistrusted. The true complexity of our lives as childless women, and the many different doors we came through to arrive in this room together, are glossed over. As are the positive and hopeful stories of women (and couples) who have not just survived this difficult experience, but moved forward in ways that feel meaningful to them.

It is absolutely vital for our sanity and sense of belonging that our stories be heard; the taboo that has kept us silent in the past needs to be dismantled one story at a time, one woman at a time. The fact that one in five women turning forty-five doesn't have children means we are hardly a minority anymore. However, whereas childfree women are beginning to be heard (they tend not to feel so self-conscious or ashamed about their situation as it was a choice), childless women are still misunderstood and misrepresented.

The power of stories is that they can recreate old worlds or create new ones. They have the ability to transform our reality, even our memories, and with that, our beliefs.

I have learned that through telling our stories to each other as childless women and then by examining some of the ways we've chosen to interpret our own (often by using some of the dominant narratives of our time – success/failure, smart/dumb choices, etc.) we can begin to shift our perspective. With support and recognition, we can let go of the feeling of being victimised by our circumstances and begin to see the benefits and opportunities they bring. (*Yeah, right*, I hear you say!) In doing so, we can create a story that makes more sense to us right now, one which supports us as we create a fulfilling and meaningful future; one that serves us and other childless women.

Stories touch us, move us, change us. Telling our stories, hearing others' stories and finally feeling heard changes us too.

Our Stories

Women who have attended my workshops or who are part of the Gateway Women online community have often told me that the experience of hearing other women's stories and sharing their own has really shifted something for them. So many of us seem to carry a disempowering version of our story in our heads, often filled with shame-based judgements about the decisions and circumstances that have contributed to our childlessness. We often say things to ourselves that we would never say (or even think) about that of another childless woman. So I wanted to recreate the experience for you of sitting in a circle of childless women as they share their experiences.

With enormous generosity and courage, some women I've come to know have trusted me with their thoughts and feelings, which you will find sprinkled throughout this book. I'd like to say thank you from the bottom of my heart to them for doing this for me, for you and for us. Names and identifying details have been changed where requested.

As you read their words, I'd like you to imagine that you are all together in a place that feels very safe to you: perhaps somewhere in nature around a campfire, far away from where anyone can hear you or see you, or maybe in a large, safe and peaceful room. You are sitting in a circle with a group of women that you've recently met, and are giving each other the gift of your full attention as you listen without interrupting, without asking questions and without offering advice . . .

Laura's Story: 47, Single (UK)

I had always dreamed of and imagined getting married and having children, but as my twenties turned into my thirties and then my forties, I found that I had not met the right guy to share my life with. I had also experienced some gynaecological issues that would have made getting pregnant slightly more challenging. I had a strong sense of having failed and I think this had a huge impact on how I felt about myself. I think those feelings came about simply because I found it so difficult to accept that what I wanted – a husband and children – appeared to be so easy for so many people around me, yet out of my grasp. Without a doubt, I thought that a partner and children would 'just happen' for me. Why wouldn't it?! I think, looking back on my experience, I should have definitely questioned the relationships with the men that I was with – it may have had something to do with not valuing myself and that manifested itself in the guys that I dated and had longer-term relationships with. But then again, other women seemed to be making similar 'mistakes' and things still 'worked out' for them . . .

Kyla's Story: 43, Married (USA)

My husband and I didn't start trying to have a child until I was thirty-six. First we tried naturally then we moved on to fertility treatments. We had two pregnancies. With the first, upon a doctor's check-up at around ten weeks, there was no longer a heartbeat. The second pregnancy went to sixteen weeks and then we got the news that the baby had Down's syndrome. We terminated the pregnancy, which was very traumatising. With the emotional turmoil and my approaching fortieth birthday, I realised that my dream of becoming a mother had come to an end.

Marianne's Story: 63, Married (UK)

I didn't start trying for a baby until my early thirties, but it didn't happen. I had always suffered from very painful periods, but had never seen a doctor about it. When we were referred to the fertility clinic, a laparoscopy confirmed the doctor's suspicion that I had quite extensive endometriosis. The suggested plan was that we have fertility treatment, which involved a few years of monthly injections, scans and pills, but no IVF, which was fairly limited on the National Health Service at that time and we were not in a financial position to pay for private treatment. As the years went by, I became more and more sad and depressed, so we made the decision to stop the treatment. I was in my forties by then. However, financially well-off friends saw my pain and offered to pay for a 'last-ditch-attempt' round of IVF. But before we could proceed, I was diagnosed with breast cancer. Following surgery, I was told that I needed an instant menopause because of the type of cancer and my risk of recurrence. I will never forget trying to tell the oncologist that I was so sad about the end of my fertility and all he said was, 'Well, it'll get rid of the endometriosis.' We considered adoption and started along that route, but we had to pull out as the process was just too hard.

Jill's Story: 45, Single (UK)

Although I wanted children, I never seemed to be in the right sort of relationship. The first real chance wasn't until my early thirties, but the guy started drinking; the next didn't want children. So then I decided to 'go it alone' with fertility treatment and for several years in my thirties and very early forties tried IUI and IVF with donor sperm eleven times, both with and without drugs. Eleven times! The result was sadly just one brief pregnancy. Then they found a polyp when I was forty-one and I decided to stop trying (I was also broke by then!). I found myself stuck in a rut with my job because I'd stayed somewhere whilst I was doing the fertility treatments, always thinking that 'very soon' I'd be pregnant as a single woman, so I needed to hang on in there for the best maternity conditions and pay I could get. After I stopped treatment at forty-one I found myself involved in a slightly mad 'limbo' type relationship, probably as a way to avoid my grief. A few years on, I'm still working through the grief, but now that I know I'm not going to be responsible for a child, my focus is on getting my working life sorted out.

Kyoko's Story: 47, Married (Japan)

I would say my childlessness results from a mixture of lack of strategy and immaturity. In short, I was reluctant to become a mother in my youth, and when I decided that I should have a try, it seemed to be too late. Yes, I belong to this particular generation that thinks you have to be independent socially, financially and emotionally. I was thirty-one years old when I got married and I was unemployed at that time. So, when I got a job, I thought that I shouldn't get pregnant until I'd been there for at least three years – it's really important that you are serious about your work in Japan. However, within two years I lost my health and so stopped working and then started a new job when I was thirty-four. After three years in *that* job I decided I was ready to get pregnant as (I thought) I had established my career. Guess what, I could not get pregnant at all! Besides, both my partner and I were too tired to have sex on week nights in our thirties and, perhaps having had enough of desperately trying to avoid pregnancy during our twenties, we'd rather gone off it! So we did our best to get pregnant with a decade of once-a-month weekend sex. (Yes, I know it wasn't enough, but we were both tired.) Years passed and I lost my job anyway due to the organisation going bankrupt. Unemployment is one of the most frightening things in Japan, where we do not have decent social housing, there's little government support for childcare costs and we only get three months of financial support (six months if you're older) from the government if you're out of work.

Liska's Story: 44, Married (Sweden)

When I was in my teens I thought that getting married and then having children would just happen when I was about twenty-five! I always wanted to have children, but I felt I needed to find the right man to build a family with. I met my husband when I was thirty-four and I thought it would be no problem getting pregnant at that age, just that it sometimes took a bit more time. But we couldn't get pregnant, so we did IVF. There wasn't anything wrong with us – we got perfect embryos from the four IVFs we did; but I wasn't able to remain pregnant with them – they just didn't stay. Instead I developed a hormonal breast tumour and I was thrown into another struggle. When I recovered from the cancer the National Board of Health and Welfare here in Sweden wouldn't allow us to adopt because of my cancer history. Not being allowed to adopt really smashed involuntary childlessness into my face, especially as I believe my breast cancer occurred as a result of going through IVF four times … I have received way more understanding and support for the cancer than the childlessness, and no one seems to be able to understand that the cancer can be cured, but that the childlessness will be with me forever …

Claude's Story: 44, Single (UK)

I always wanted to be a mother and have a family of my own. It was a dream I had. I was in what I thought was a stable and long-lasting relationship. We both wanted a family. But being two women, this was never going to be easy. We had emigrated to a country where being in a same-sex relationship made no difference whatsoever to having fertility treatment and we were surrounded by people who'd done exactly that. Through eight treatments of IUI I got pregnant twice, a year apart. Unfortunately, I lost both my babies to miscarriage at exactly the same time of year. The grief was immense and took a toll on both of us. My partner then left me for another woman, someone much older with teenage kids. So my dream went up in smoke and, whilst I dealt with the divorce and the legal fallout from that thousands of miles from home, I buried the grief for my childlessness as deep as I could. I just didn't have the energy to deal with being childless too. It's only in the last two or three years that I have started to uncover the grief that comes with being childless.

Delia's Story: 48, Living with Partner (UK)

I met my future husband when I was twenty – very young but I thought I knew what I wanted and that I was a grown-up woman. He swept me off my feet and I moved to Greece to live with him – a gorgeous Greek god who turned out to be a very controlling, violent man. I stayed because it seemed easier somehow – I was a long way from home and to get on a plane was to admit that it wasn't working, first to myself and then to my family and friends. We got married – it was easier than leaving. Deep down I knew that it wouldn't be the right thing to do to have children with him and my body seemed to know that too as I had a stress-induced hormone imbalance that made it difficult for me to become pregnant. I finally got the courage to leave in my late twenties and it took the next ten years – my most fertile years – for me to get over my experience. I met my current partner when we were both in our forties. We talked about starting a family but decided that it was far too late to be having our own children: he has three grown-up children already. He has been the stable, loving relationship I had been craving all my life and being with him has given me the strength to work through the grief of my childlessness, as well as the overwhelming emotions that I feel along the way as I come to terms with what happened to me and the domestic abuse I experienced.

EXERCISE 1
Your Story

Now it's your turn to tell your story in the circle of childless women. I'd like you to imagine that you are sitting with us and, having listened to all of the other women's stories with respectful attention, compassion and understanding, and having observed them do the same, you now feel able to share yours. You can do so in your mind, say it out loud or write it down – whatever feels possible for you right now.

Your story is now part of *our* story. Another precious piece in the mosaic of childlessness. Welcome to your tribe.

Reflections on Chapter 1

Take a moment to reflect on how the last week has been for you, or however long it's been since you worked through Chapter 1. Have you noticed any new thoughts and feelings coming up?

I didn't realise when I very first started sharing my own story on my blog in 2011 what a powerful thing I was doing – I didn't realise that being open and honest about my childlessness, and all the twists and turns that led up to it, was breaking a social taboo. I just had to share my truth in the desperate hope that someone, even just one person, would read it, and I would no longer be alone with it. The burden of my story was too much for me to carry any longer; I needed to put it down. However, what surprised me was that by sharing my story I somehow gave permission for many other women to share theirs too, and the exchange of healing began. Often, as happened for me on my blog, what I see in Gateway Women workshops and groups is that we recognise elements of *our* story in another woman's, which helps us feel less freakish and ashamed and encourages us to risk the vulnerability of opening up. Hearing that others have experienced similar heartbreaks, reversals of fortune, bad luck, unfortunate timings and have made what, in retrospect, seem like 'stupid' decisions helps to normalise our history. We are no longer alone. Even if the details are different (and we *are* all different), the ending of the story is one we all share, and often some of the plot twists too. There is great relief to be found in not being alone with it any more. And knowing too that it's safe in the hearts and minds of others, because they understand at a very personal level how private, precious and painful this story is.

So, how was it for you to sit in the imaginary circle with these brave childless women and hear their stories, some of the thousands I've heard over the past few years?

- Did you notice any threads between some of their stories and your own, and how does that feel?

- Did you find it easier to be understanding and compassionate towards them and their stories than you are towards yourself about your own? Does that seem fair?

- Which factors from the 'Fifty Ways Not to Be a Mother' list on pages 20–4 connect to *your* story?

- Can you sense that it may be possible now to soften some of the harshness you might feel towards yourself for how things turned out? As you've heard, the reasons for being childless are never simple, and much of what happened was outside our control, no matter how much we torture ourselves with 'what ifs'.

So many of us are carrying so much shame attached to our stories, but when we hear others tell theirs and begin to notice that we don't automatically think badly of *them* for how things turned out, we begin to consider easing up on ourselves. And once the energy formerly used in beating ourselves up starts going towards healing and growing ... well, it creates a space for new things to start happening. It doesn't matter how small the shift is, it's the start that matters. It's like the 'trim tab', that small flap on the rudder of an ocean liner or an aeroplane wing which moves first, and in doing so creates a tiny change in flow that makes possible a big change in direction.

Small changes can have a very big effect!

Life is
LONG,
but
fertility is
SHORT.

CHAPTER 2

You're Not Alone

It's been my experience, and confirmed by the many women I've worked with, that placing your own story within a broader framework can help you to begin to view it in a new light. You can have fresh thoughts, make new connections, have 'aha' moments and perhaps even begin to turn the volume down on that track in your head that says, *It's all your fault* ...

So in this chapter, we're going to take a closer look at both the cultural context within which your own childlessness takes place, as well as your early childhood experiences and what you learned from them about dating, mating and motherhood.

Although when you look around you in the street, amongst your friends and family or in the media you may sometimes feel like the *only* woman who isn't a mother, the surprising fact is that around one in five women have reached their mid-forties without having had children.[3] So where the hell are they all then?

> *The numbers certainly make me feel less of a freak, although my Facebook feed continues to do so.*
>
> Sarah: 45, Single, USA

If you think about it, mothers are fairly easy to spot because they either have children with them, or may be sporting some of the identifying accessories of modern motherhood, such as a baby seat in the back of their car or a cute picture of them as a screensaver on their phone, and even if none of these things are visible, they'll be quite likely to bring their children into the conversation fairly soon. But childless women are not so easily identified and indeed many childless women know other childless women and yet can go for decades without mentioning it, for fear of embarrassing them. It's possible to find ourselves feeling very alone, when in fact we have childless sisters in our midst. Although of course this can vary from urban to rural settings, and may also depend on your social circle. I didn't know any at all.

> *I've recently realised that I have many childless female friends and colleagues (I did a quick headcount and could name ten instantly; there may be more). And yet neither before nor after joining Gateway Women have I discussed this issue with them.*
>
> Natasha: 53, Single, UK

The last time the rate of childlessness was this high in the population was for women born around 1900. Research has shown that this was due to two factors: the large number of women who remained unmarried due to the loss of so many men in the First World War, and the effect of the Great Depression of the 1930s on both fertility and finances.[4] Rather shockingly these were known as the 'surplus women'.[5]

The fact that it took the most devastating war this world has seen in terms of loss of life, coupled with the Great Depression, to suppress birth rates to the same extent as now, shows that we are indeed living through a period of massive social change. It really isn't 'just us'.

Childlessness Around the World[6]

To put childlessness into a global context, the 2013 United Nations Fertility Report states that since the UN's 1994 International Conference on Population and Development, the number of low-fertility countries (with 2.0 children per woman or fewer) has increased from 51 to 70. Within those countries, childlessness amongst women aged 40–44 has increased across Europe and Eastern Asia, with five countries now having 1 in 5 women remaining childless, a statistic unknown in 1994.[7]

> *UK and Ireland:* According to the UK Office for National Statistics, 20 per cent of women born between 1961 and 1966 remain without children, dropping slightly to 19 per cent for those born in 1967. The most recent 'completed childbearing' data available, for those born in 1968, drops again to 18 per cent. However, this is still *double* the 11 per cent of their mothers' generation. From speaking to many childless women born in the 1970s, I think it's quite likely that this may grow to 25 per cent of women because of the combined impact of 'social infertility' (being unable to find a suitable partner), along with delaying or not feeling able to have children for financial reasons due to the global economic downturn since 2008. The data available so far shows that up to 47 per cent of women born in the 1970s were childless at the age of thirty, compared to up to 28 per cent of their mothers' generation, which may be one such early sign.[8] Ireland's rate of childlessness is similarly 18 per cent for those born in 1965.[9]

> *USA:* Almost 20 per cent of women remained childless by the mid-2000s, but this number dropped to 15 per cent in 2014. Some analysis predicts that childbearing delayed due to the global economic downturn may prove to be 'fertility foregone', but it is too early to tell for sure.[10] This compares to data from the mid-1970s, which showed that 10 per cent of women were childless.[11] The childbearing rate of women in their twenties fell 15 per cent

between 2007 and 2012 and it remains to be seen how many of these 'Millennials' go on to have children in their thirties and early forties.[12]

Canada: Almost 19 per cent of Canadian women were childless aged 40–44 in 2011, more than double the previously recorded rate in 1992.[13] Also, according to the 2011 census,[14] there are now more people living in single-person households than households with children.[15] The same survey also shows that 44.5 per cent of Canadian couples are 'without children'.[16]

Australia and New Zealand: In Australia, 24 per cent of women of childbearing age are expected to remain childless. This compares to 9 per cent for women born between 1930 and 1946, who benefited from the improved economic outlook after World War II.[17] In New Zealand, 25 per cent of women born in 1975 are expected to remain childless, compared to 10 per cent of women aged 44–49 in its 2006 survey, and 9 per cent in 1981.[18]

Europe: France[19] and Sweden[20] have two of the lowest rates of childlessness (due to liberal state support for working mothers and families) at 10 per cent and 13 per cent,[21] whilst Germany has the highest rate at 28 per cent,[22] with Italy coming in second at 24 per cent[23] and then Spain at almost 22 per cent.[24] Some of the other European countries with a high rate of childlessness (around 20 per cent) are Austria, Finland and the Netherlands.[25]

East Asia: In Japan, of those women born in the 1960s, almost 13 per cent have no children. However, for those born in the 1970s, it is expected that 30 per cent (almost 1 in 3) will remain childless.[26] Singapore has the highest current rate of childlessness amongst women aged 40–44, at 23 per cent (almost 1 in 4).[27] According to the UN report, East Asia would appear to be the area where childlessness is growing most quickly.[28]

Your Story in Context: the Shock-Absorber Generation

I call those of us born in the 1960s and 1970s to mothers who hadn't had the same easy access to birth control, higher education and professional careers that we did the 'shock-absorber generation for the sexual revolution'.

My mother, who'd had me at eighteen 'out of wedlock' (as it was called in those days), married unhappily whilst I was still a toddler in order to provide a 'respectable' home for me. As I grew up, she instilled in me the belief that a life *outside* the domestic sphere was the one to aspire to, and that education and ambition were the way to achieve that.

Now, I'm not saying that *every* 1960s and 1970s mother would have given the same message, but I've spoken to enough childless women aged forty and over to know that many of us can identify with this. However, like all aspects of circumstantial childlessness, a great deal more research needs to be done.

> *My mother often made comments along the lines of, 'If I had to do it again, I would not have had children.' At the same time, she also mentions all the pregnancies of my childhood friends, makes negative comments about childless women and complains about our small family. Her comments totally confused me.*
>
> Sarah: 45, Single, USA

Although the contraceptive pill was made available on the NHS (the British National Health Service) in 1961,[29] my Catholic-raised mother knew so little about how babies were made that she didn't even know she needed to use contraception, and hence my unscheduled arrival in 1964.

Whilst my mother never told me *not* to have children, she made it pretty clear that there were other options that were *more* interesting, meaningful and liberating for me to aspire to. When I became sexually active as a teenager, she encouraged me to go on the Pill immediately. She also taught me the facts of life so early (I think I was about eight) that I really didn't have a clue what she was talking about! Her love for me included protecting me from what had happened to her.

> When I was growing up, my mum always seemed very busy, and had no time for us as children, often saying how tired she was. When I was a teenager there was never any real discussion about having children, what to expect or even if I wanted them. The only thing I remember was a conversation as a teenager – I must have been talking about boys, etc., and Mum said, 'Right, you're going on the Pill. I don't want any unwanted babies in this house!' No discussion, no explanation about what she meant. It put the fear of God in me not to become pregnant and for a long time I felt that children were something people 'endured', that they got in the way, that they were a burden.
>
> Delia: 48, Living with Partner, UK

Perhaps men who've grown up with similarly frustrated mothers also picked up that having a family 'traps' you. This, reinforced by the fact that women don't need the kind of financial support they used to, may have contributed to some men feeling that they don't have to make early and long-term commitments. If women can have children out of marriage and it's no longer a 'sin'; if you don't *have* to marry a woman if you get her pregnant; and if sex doesn't automatically run the risk of pregnancy, where's the urgency for men to settle down these days? They can remain 'free' for as long as they want and many are choosing to do so. There's also not the same status to being a 'family man' that there once was – these days it seems that a high disposable income and a good-looking partner bring more kudos than the more private sacrifices and satisfactions of family and domestic life.

Perhaps some men are also reluctant to take on the role of fatherhood having seen so little of their *own* fathers whilst growing up.

Combined with his frustrated mother's possible resentment towards her own subservient role and the unspoken (or spoken) resentment she had towards his father, it's not hard to imagine that he might wish to construct his life on an entirely different template.

The old 'marriage deal' isn't really possible anymore and its prevalence in the past may actually have been overstated in our current cultural longing for more 'settled' times. Those sole-breadwinner families living in comfortably sized homes maintained by a secure income may not have actually existed in the numbers that our nostalgia believes, and they certainly hardly exist anymore, except for the extremely well-off. Meanwhile, back in the real world, professionals such as teachers, solicitors and doctors, many of whom in the past were able to afford to support their families on one income, now scrabble to achieve something like it on two, whilst suffering from not enough sleep and accruing a mountain of debt.

> *I would have liked the option to be a stay-at-home mother (and would have preferred that to working full-time) but I think that 1950s lifestyle was probably an anomaly and we would do better by women to emulate countries like Sweden and France, where they make it easier for women to both have children and work. The dirty secret is that if women were guaranteed an attractive, responsible, loving partner who would support them for life, most would probably be perfectly happy to stay home and raise a family (of course there would still be a small percentage who would want a career). But life has never offered that guarantee, and there have always been miserable marriages in which women have been trapped. For their own security, women need to be able to support themselves.*
>
> Sarah: 45, Single, USA

The next generation, growing up in such stressed-out families and watching their parents tear themselves (and possibly each other) apart trying to make it work, will probably choose a very different model to organise *their* own family lives. But the shock-absorber generation?

We're the ones metabolising these changes into our culture, and many of us are reeling from the disparity between our lives and the ones we *expected* to be living. And sadly many of us think that's our own fault – and that's certainly the message that mainstream culture reflects back at us.

Since humans evolved, if men and women were having sex, it was quite likely that it would lead to a baby at some point. It's important to realise what a complete and absolute game-changer the Pill has been in all our lives.

The sexual revolution has enabled women to achieve increased equality in many areas, but not in terms of fertility. Life is long but fertility is short and, as so many of us tried to pack education, career, marriage and babies into our twenties and thirties (with a last dash to the altar of the fertility gods in our early forties), the disparity between men's and women's fertility has become clearer than ever.

Women have joined a professional working world which has grown up around the male template of working incredibly hard to establish your career in your twenties and thirties and to delay starting a family – a model which runs counter to female fertility. Sadly, this is something that many of us who are childless-by-circumstance have found out the hard way.

My mother impressed upon me that you have to get a good education and a job before you get pregnant. That you have to be successful if you want to be a mother in order to be financially independent, because, if you divorce, fathers tend to pay the child support only for two years. And so, when I asked my mom what the point was of having children, she said, 'You could learn tolerance.' Is that all, I thought? These days I can see that learning tolerance from your kids wouldn't be so bad, but at the time I was unimpressed.

Kyoko: 47, Married, Japan

In 2012, University of Huddersfield psychologist Kirsty Budds ana-lysed the media rhetoric around 'delayed motherhood' and concluded that:

> For a lot of women it isn't a selfish choice but is based around careful decisions, careful negotiations and life circumstances such as the right partner and the right financial position. These women are effectively responsibly trying to produce the best situation in which to have children, which is encouraged societally, but then they are chastised because they are giving birth when older, when it is more risky.[30]

The Pill, women's education, and women's wholesale entry into higher education and the professional working world has completely changed the way men and women relate to each other socially, cultur-ally, sexually and as potential parents.

In one generation, we've turned on their head aeons of courtship and mating behaviours, and we're still working this through within the day-to-day context of our lives. We're a living experiment.

Men too are finding it 'harder to be a man today than it was in their fathers' generation', and looking at how the changes in women's lives have affected them is slowly becoming an area of legitimate academic study.[31]

Hopefully, the generations that come after us will learn from our experiment that 'having it all' is a myth and that equality should mean that both men *and* women are *equally* entitled to live in a culture that makes it possible to live balanced, healthy and purposeful lives, whether that involves being a parent or not.

Choice, What Choice?

In 1969, Carol Hanisch's paper 'The Personal is Political'[32] was published and remains a key text today within the feminist movement. And yet here we are, almost half a century later, fighting for the choice to be mothers.

'Failing' to become a mother, particularly when there are no obvious medical issues, is seen primarily as some kind of 'choice'. Yet for those of us who've lived that choice, we know that it's a damned-if-you-do, damned-if-you-don't kind of choice, for example:

- What choice is it to choose to become a mother with a man you're not sure is going to stick around?
- What choice is it to choose to become a single or partnered mother in a society where childcare can cost almost your whole salary?
- What choice is it to put off motherhood until you (and your partner) can afford it, but risk age-related infertility?
- And so on ...

Most women I've spoken to feel that their 'failure' to become a mother is because of the 'poor choices' *they've* made and that they should have made different choices, for example:

- That she should have married 'him', even though she wasn't sure she really loved him.
- That she shouldn't have married 'him' because he was always a bit flaky.
- That she should have started internet dating earlier.
- That she should have got pregnant 'accidentally on purpose'.
- That she should have had the baby she conceived at twenty.

- That she should have educated herself about her fertility much, much earlier.

- That she should have been more adventurous, or more cautious.

- That she should have frozen her eggs.

- And so on ...

The list is endless.

'Should' is an exhausting, finger-wagging word which reaffirms one of the dominant beliefs of our time – that everything in life is down to making the *right choices*. With such a belief driving you, your list of 'should haves' is one you can rake over indefinitely. And that way lies madness ...

These are rock-and-a-hard-place choices that fail to take into account the wider socio-cultural environment, one which includes, for example, the choices that our potential partners in parenthood are making for themselves in their thirties and forties; the effects of archaic educational and working patterns and employment insecurity; the incredibly high cost of living in many developed countries; a widespread ignorance of the high failure rate of IVF (around 75 per cent[33]); and governments that bang on about 'hard-working families' without funding simple, practical measures that would make parenthood more affordable and egalitarian.

It's also time that the feminist movement took serious notice of the prejudiced position of childless and childfree women in our society. A good deal of the focus of first- and second-wave feminism was on a woman's right to choose when to have children, to provide access to legalised and safe abortion and to support their rights as working mothers. All of this was, and is, hugely important, and much of this battle remains to be won, particularly in developing countries. However, it's now time to broaden the feminist agenda to include the experience of those of us who have either chosen or haven't been able to become mothers and to look at how and why we are undermined, undervalued and disempowered as women as a result. It came as a huge shock to me, having been brought up to be independent, to earn my own living and to consider myself a man's equal, to find myself invisibly sidelined in my forties by men, and also by many mothers.

The Swedish Way

The kind of environment that supports women (and men) in their choice to parent is *not* economically impossible, despite what many governments say. They've done it in Sweden and reversed the European-wide post-baby-boom drop in birth rates, whilst simultaneously increasing the number of working women. Sweden has an almost equal number of men and women in the workforce, more women on the boards of top companies than in any other country and an equality in the domestic tasks of childrearing unknown elsewhere in the developed world. The result: an egalitarian and highly productive economy.[34] However, it still doesn't make it easy to be a childless woman; in some ways it might even be harder, given the government support all around you making all kind of motherhood options (including solo motherhood) possible, such as state-funded IVF treatments, generous maternity leave benefits and high-quality state-funded childcare. Perhaps it might make you feel even more like an oddball! Indeed, Liska said, 'in Sweden, nobody talks about it at all. That's why I felt so alone when I ended up being childless. I wanted to talk to someone who would tell me that life was going to be OK, but there wasn't anyone, nor any websites or blogs in Swedish. Luckily I found some in English.'

So how did Sweden achieve this feat of social engineering? By ensuring that time off when a baby is born is generous *and* making it a requirement that it be shared equally between both parents; by making high-quality, state-provided childcare freely available and providing excellent state education and healthcare. Yes, they pay for it with a 56.6 per cent rate of income tax, but consider it fair and well spent.[35] Indeed, in a speech given to the UN and the World Bank in July 2015, the Swedish Prime Minister, Stefan Löfven, said, 'Gender equality is not only morally right. It is also an extremely potent development and growth booster.'[36]

The French Way

In France, 'family-friendly' policies have had a dramatic effect on restoring the birth-rate slump after the post-war baby boom. However, what is interesting is that the *type* of family the French state supports is *not* the classic nuclear family, but a much more fluid and modern one, filled with 'late marriages, reconstituted families, single parents, [and] much more frequent births outside marriage'.[37] In other words, the type of family that more accurately reflects life in developed countries.

What the French state also provides help for is the very thing that traditionalists feared would reduce birth rates most; offering support for mothers in the workplace, allowing them financially and practically to be able to remain in work. Through providing state-subsidised childcare, creating a business and service culture where not every child-related appointment happens at 3.30 p.m.,[38] and de-stigmatising the role of 'working mother'[39] France keeps its birth rate high and its childlessness rate low. Compare this to the UK, where in a populist newspaper a headline such as 'Working mothers risk damaging their child's prospects'[40] is quite common.[41]

Nonetheless, despite the seemingly egalitarian nature of the French system, it still supports a very 'traditional' role of mothers, as it seems that their 'family-friendly' policies are heavily weighted towards supporting mothers, whilst fathers are mostly left out of the picture, receiving just eleven days of paid paternity leave, compared to sixteen weeks for mothers (twenty-six weeks if a third child).[42] Thus, traditional gender roles are still tacitly supported, and this shows in the fact that there are comparatively few women in senior management positions, and even fewer elected female representative in Parliament (20 per cent as opposed to the OECD norm of 25 per cent).[43]

The Rest of Us

So, it is possible to support women to be able to afford to have children, and also to provide affordable childcare that enables them to both work and bring up their children. But it's expensive. Both Sweden and France spend 3.5 per cent of their GDP on such benefits and 'the map of fertility rates in the EU is remarkably similar to that of childcare facilities'.[44] However, for those of us who wanted to have children, not being able to afford them is a reason that, although it undoubtedly has an impact, would appear to be far from the most common factor.

The number of adults ageing without children is a concern in those countries with a high rate of childlessness, with Japan[45] most readily coming to mind, although recent estimates show that in the UK too at least 20 per cent of adults (men and women) currently in their forties will be ageing without children.[46] An economic model that is based on the younger generation paying for elderly people's needs doesn't really work in 'low-fertility' countries, and it's presenting such societies with a big logistical headache. Headlines such as 'Trend of couples not having children just plain selfish'[47] (which is sadly a common refrain, both in private conversations and in the press) doesn't help. What perhaps some people fail to recognise is that possibly only 10 per cent of childless women actively chose not to be mothers.[48] And trying to 'shame' us isn't going to do anything to help raise the birth rate, or it probably would have already worked ...

I'll be exploring both the fears and possibilities around ageing without children in Chapter 12. Bet you can't wait!

Messages and Choices

Grab a pile of Post-it notes or some small pieces of paper. Use them to write down individual words or phrases that come to mind in response to this exercise.

Spend a few minutes thinking about some of the 'messages' you picked up about dating, mating, marrying and mothering when you were a child. It might be the kinds of things that significant adults said to you, but it might also include inferences you made having witnessed the way that certain people or situations were talked about (or silenced) in your home. It might also include the prevailing cultural messages that may have filtered through to you from your local community, school, church, the media, etc.

Here are some examples that others have come up with doing this exercise:

- Get an education and see the world first.
- If you're not engaged by the time you're thirty, you're on the shelf.
- Motherhood is every woman's destiny.
- Being a mother is a thankless task.
- Children ruin your life.
- Without children, you're not a real woman.
- Marriage before baby carriage.
- Nice girls finish last.
- Childless 'career women' are pitiful.
- Always be financially independent.
- Once you've had a child you're trapped.
- Without a baby you're not complete.

- If you don't have kids, you'll always regret it.
- If you do have kids, you'll always regret it!
- And so on ...

Once you've written them out, stick them on a window or mirror and step back to take a look at them all together.

- Do they make coherent sense as a whole, or do some of them contradict each other?
- Do you still believe these are 'facts' or can you see they might be just opinions, and perhaps not even *your* opinions?
- Reflect on which messages still feel congruent with the person you are today and which ones are past their sell-by date.
- Using this information, reflect on the notion that your 'choices' around relationships and having a family may not have been entirely 'free choices' after all ...

Reflections on Chapter 2

In this chapter we've taken a galloping tour through the socio-economic and cultural background to the largest increase in childlessness since the First World War and the Great Depression combined. We've looked at the growth of childlessness across the developed world and some of the ways that societies are tackling it. We've even touched on ageing without children and the demographic headache this is creating. And then, to top it all, you've taken a look at how helpful or unhelpful some of the messages from your childhood have been in shaping your conscious and subconscious thoughts about becoming or not becoming a mother.

And now ... breathe!

You may be wondering, what's all this about? How does all this relate to *my* pain, *my* confusion, *my* fears, *my* hopes, *my* childlessness? This isn't the kind of thing I was expecting in this book ...

However, I hope that you've found that starting to view your own story in a new way, both from a personal perspective (your own childhood experience) and also within a broader cultural one, has helped you to look at things differently. It's also possible that some of these new realisations might make you feel angry when you realise that your choices (the very ones you've beaten yourself up about for so very long) were perhaps not entirely your own to make, nor the consequences of them quite so much your fault as you, and others, sometimes insist. And yet at other times, knowing that you were not quite the free agent of modernity that you had believed can bring you some relief. It's also possible to feel both angry and relieved at the same time!

If you did the 'Messages and Choices' exercise, you may have noticed that quite a few of the 'beliefs' you hold (or held) about being a woman, being a mother, about men, relationships, careers, etc., were often contradictory and that you probably don't even agree with half of them anymore, if you ever fully did. Sometimes it can come as quite a surprise to us when we realise how much credence we've given to messages that, although they may have made some sense to us when we were kids (or that we trusted would make sense when we grew up), have remained unexamined and thus active, to this day. Although you may be profoundly upset and full of regret to realise that some of your major life decisions have been strongly influenced by beliefs your adult self disagrees with, this is not another reason to give yourself a hard time. What it *does* mean is that from this point forward, you have the option to choose your beliefs consciously and with great care.

Lifting the lid on your familial and cultural conditioning can be quite unnerving. You may feel a bit rattled, and that's to be expected. You may notice new thoughts and feelings, even dreams, as you digest the contents of this chapter. It can take time for this all to 'percolate' through your memories and awareness.

Whatever you find yourself doing, be gentle with yourself whilst you make space in your inner world for this broader view.

LIFE
can be tough.

MOTHERHOOD
can be tough.

CHILDLESSNESS
can be tough.

CHAPTER 3

Motherhood with a Capital 'M'

Being a Mother Means …

How do you mentally finish that sentence in your mind? Does it include any of the following?

- Love
- Nurturing
- Comfort
- Play
- Never being alone
- Grandchildren
- Laughter
- Cuddles
- Fulfilment
- Being a real woman
- And so on …

Whilst such things are commonly associated with the joy of motherhood in our culture, for many of us who have been denied that experience, we may erroneously come to believe that many of them are *only* accessible through motherhood.

It isn't true, but it's an overwhelming cultural belief right now. Everywhere you look, motherhood with a capital 'M' is trumpeted as the answer to absolutely everything. This isn't helpful to mothers either, as it makes it very hard for them to be open and honest about how tough and unsatisfying motherhood can be sometimes.

The good news is that there *are* other ways to access many of the experiences and feelings that you currently associate only with motherhood. Right now, you may be suspicious of this suggestion, but please stay with me! Whilst the experience of being a mother has a uniquely intense quality that we will never know, it is absolutely *not* the only way to access joy, fulfilment, meaning, love, play and many of the other things you might currently feel deprived of.

Motherhood is not an inoculation against sadness, disappointment, ageing, loss, abandonment, betrayal, disease, old age and death.

The human condition is a struggle for us all – a mixture of joy and sadness, of getting or not getting what we want and losing those things we care about. This is true for all of us, mothers or not.

> *I spent way too many years feeling that joy and meaning would never be a part of my life, but I have found that by acknowledging and working with my deep creativity, I can have joy and meaning in a very fulfilling way. Gradually, these feelings are growing stronger as I allow myself to experience joy without feeling guilty about it.*
>
> Marianne: 63, Married, UK

One of my favourite sayings is often attributed to the ancient Greek philosopher Plato: 'Be kind. For everyone you meet is fighting a hard battle.'[49]

> *Having children is not a free pass to a happy life. If we look at the lives of mothers without envy and listen to them without prejudice, we know this to be true. They suffer too and sometimes their children are the very source of that suffering.*

In fact, Rachel Cusk, who wrote a frank memoir of motherhood, *A Life's Work: On Becoming a Mother*,[50] was vilified for breaking the 'motherhood is meaningful' script. In a 2008 article for the *Guardian* she reflected on the personal and vicious mauling she received:

> These days I have a better understanding of the intolerance to which, for a while, I fell victim. I see that, like all intolerance, it arose from dependence on an ideal. I see that cruelty and rudeness and viciousness are its harbingers, as they have always been. I see that many – most – of my female detractors continue to write routinely in the press about motherhood and issues relating to children. Their interest in these issues has a fixated quality, compared with their worldly male equivalents.[51]

I remind myself to hold on to mothers who tell the truth like Rachel Cusk when other mothers tell me I'm so 'lucky' I don't have children because I get to travel, sleep in, go out late, do what I want and socialise all the time. In their minds, it's as if we childless women are still irresponsible, carefree twenty-somethings rather than the mature women with serious responsibilities and hefty financial requirements that we are.

They perhaps don't realise either that for those of us who are single, we get no tax breaks, have no one to split the bills with and rarely have anything left over at the end of the month with which to socialise and go on holidays. Indeed, in January 2013, *The Atlantic* magazine published a detailed analysis by Lisa Arnold and Christina Campbell called 'The High Price of Being Single in America',[52] showing their calculations that over a lifetime, being a single woman (as compared to a married one) costs between $484,368 and $1,022,096 extra. *'More than a million dollars just for being single,'* they wrote. Later in the same article the authors claimed that they had 'made only the most conservative of estimates' because they too thought that 'these sums are just too crazy: surely we must have miscalculated or reasoned wrong'.

It seems that even those living the reality of being single (as both the authors of the article were) found their analysis of the data hard to believe because it went against the established belief that single childless women have both money and time to burn and really nothing to moan about.

I have understanding friends with kids. But only other nomos (particularly those who are single) can really grasp the implications of being outside the framework of motherhood and/or a lifelong partnership. It's going to affect you at every stage of your life.

Kim: 43, Single, France/UK

We know that the 'rich and carefree' fantasy that parents have about childless adults isn't true (well, not for most of us anyway), so perhaps we can begin to see that *our* fantasies about the lives of parents may be similarly unreal. Rachel Cusk is one of the very few mothers who has dared to tell the truth of her experience of motherhood to those 'not in the know', yet these are matters which many mothers share freely with each other in private. It was not *what* Cusk said, but *who* she said it to that seemed to be the problem. I look forward to the day when we succeed in dismantling the whole 'mummy myth' so that mothers-to-be know what to *really* expect when they're expecting and childless women are not made miserable with the idea that they are only allowed the scraps of life.

I really suffered from the pronatalist message that not having children will always be the 'second-best option'. There are hardly any positive stories in the media of women who wanted to have children but couldn't. Generally the stories are about women who never gave up and then had children, or who devoted their lives to charitable causes in place of becoming a mother.

Heather: 40, Married, UK

The fetishisation of motherhood is a fantasy that serves neither mothers nor nomos and oppresses both. It also divides women in such a way as to serve the status quo by keeping us squabbling and suspicious of each other, rather than supporting each other as we move forward to full equality.

As childless women, part of our journey back to a full and happy life again is beginning to see the whole picture, not just the glossy media fantasy of motherhood. Life can be tough. Motherhood can be tough. Childlessness can be tough.

However, whereas the trials of motherhood are, on the surface, recognised and understood by others, the trials of childlessness often seem to be completely invisible and deemed worthless. For all the kindness and empathy we childless women show others around us; for all the understanding and support we give to the mothers in our lives and communities; for all the talk about children and childrearing we sit through politely, unable to contribute to – sometimes it seems that the only ones who have any concept of the compromises, difficulties and losses of our *own* lives are other childless women. Sometimes it can feel like everyone else seems to think we're either making a fuss about nothing or that we're actually really lucky not to have children but are too stupid or pathetic to notice.

What I would like is for the important people in my life to listen (without interrupting with their own agenda!) and really acknowledge that my life has not actually been the blissful existence of their imaginings. I would like them to see that I am actually really

strong to have kept standing up each time life knocked me for six.
And that it was bloody hard to keep doing that with all the dis-
missive, patronising, shaming, demeaning, mocking, humiliating,
isolating, hurtful and crushing messages we receive from the world
around us.

Jenni: 40, Single, Australia

Such lack of empathy or compassion can also be hard to bear when, on a daily basis, we see the impact of women who, whilst they were physically able to bear a child, are not psychologically mature enough, well enough or supported enough to parent. Whereas we childless women are seen as a bit of an embarrassment, frankly. Leftover women. And this can make our situation feel even worse.

For the Greeks and the Romans exile was considered a fate worse than death, because it involved being cut off from the support of friends, family and civilisation. Sometimes, being a childless woman can feel like that. Like being an unwanted stranger in your own land, not being quite sure what you did wrong to deserve this shaming, this othering.

The Fetishisation of Motherhood

For those of us who wanted to be mothers, it can seem that the whole world has gone absolutely motherhood-mad. When I was growing up in the 1970s, motherhood seemed to be a pretty 'normal' activity for women and nobody made a big deal about it. There were no design-er buggies, no glamorous children's clothes and no 'celebrity bump watch'. The grown-ups did grown-up things, ate grown-up food and seemed to have access to a grown-up world, whilst we children did chores to earn our pocket money and were often told to leave the grown-ups alone. Pregnant women wore maternity smocks to hide their bump, not figure-hugging clothes to show it off.

There was nothing noteworthy or celebratory about being pregnant outside the family circle; if anything, the impression I got as a child was that being pregnant was one of those slightly embarrassing things that women's bodies did and which you didn't talk about.

> *Motherhood has become fashionable and hence marketable in a way that has never been seen before. With that comes a whole host of forgivable transgressions. After all ... if you're 'doing the most difficult job in the world', how could you possibly wear anything but a set of wings and a shiny halo?*
>
> Alizabeth: 41, Married, Australia

Fast-forward to the twenty-first century, and we find a large swathe of (mostly) middle-class women for whom motherhood has become an unattainable dream due to 'social infertility' (not finding a suitable partner) as well as an unaffordable luxury for many couples. And our cultural response? To fetishise the trappings of motherhood.

From designer buggies to the cult of the yummy mummy and her terrifying American cousin, the 'momzilla',[53] as the writer Jill Kargmen termed her, many of today's middle-class children appear to be treated like precious and breakable artefacts and motherhood seems to have become a competitive and rarefied sport. This is not helpful for mothers, children, wider society or the future.

Whatever can be going on culturally when anyone in the public eye can make the front cover of a magazine simply for getting pregnant? It seems that right now, becoming a mother is the most noteworthy and prestigious thing a woman can do.

Now, motherhood is indeed the most important role to that woman's children, and parenting has a crucial role to play in society as the route through which the rules and beliefs of our culture are passed on. But it is not fundamentally newsworthy or miraculous. Except at Christmas – a festival celebrating the ultimate miracle baby story!

The current cultural adulation of motherhood, at a time when somewhere between one in five and one in three women are reaching the menopause without having had children, is particularly hard on childless women. It's a role that we will never be able to play and are also not considered to have a say in. A whole new generation is being reared to inhabit and inherit our world and we are expected to have no part in it, or influence over it.

The glorification of motherhood can be explained as what happens when rampant pronatalism meets rampant consumerism.

If 'pronatalism' is a new term to you (it was to me), it's explained by Laura Carroll in her 2012 book *The Baby Matrix* as:

> the idea that parenthood and raising children should be the central focus of every person's adult life. Pronatalism is a strong social force and includes a collection of beliefs so embedded that they have come to be seen as 'true'.[54]

As Carroll explores, pronatalism is not a new concept – it's been around whenever it has suited the Church, the state or the powers-that-be that expanding the population would cement its power. Even as recently as February 2015, Pope Francis said in a general address in St Peter's Square that, 'The choice to not have children is selfish.'[55]

But what *is* hard to stomach is that whilst pronatalism is being preached from pulpits and the front pages of magazines, there is little political will to create a society that would make it easier for more women to have those children if they could or wished to. I was staggered when I found out that the US, as perhaps the most rampantly pronatalist culture at present, makes no provision whatsoever for paid maternity leave. None. Zero.

One dictionary definition of 'fetish' describes it as 'an object of unreasonably excessive attention or reverence', and also 'an object that is believed to have magical or spiritual powers'. Combining pronatalism with consumerism and the rise in involuntary childlessness would appear to have turned motherhood, children and the trappings of both into a fetish. However, not all cultures are pronatalist – in Germany, the promotion of motherhood still carries a whiff of Nazi eugenics ...

The 'fetishisation of motherhood' is almost non-existent in
Germany, as it would bring back memories of Nazism. If the topic
does comes up, I find it very disturbing that childlessness is always
depicted as a conscious decision, never something one might not
have control over at all times. Moreover, this 'decision' is always
connected to utter selfishness. However, when reading the British
or American press, I notice a strange contradiction: childless/
childfree women (men don't seem to come under the same scrutiny)
are portrayed as somewhat sinister career women or, at the min-
imum, to have utterly ulterior motives, whilst stay-at-home mums
are lazy, either sponging off social services or their hard-working
husbands, or even worse, are 'Baby Mamas', living off a wealthy
or famous boyfriend.

Selda: 47, Single, Germany

A pronatalist culture is also, ironically, a hard one for mothers too, who are only able to share with each other behind closed doors the struggles and disappointments of their lives. In public, all they are 'allowed' to say is that motherhood is 'the most fulfilling thing I've ever done'.

It is summed up for me in a horrid family cafe near where my
sister lives in Holland – pink everywhere. This grotesque carica-
ture of femininity with its cupcakes and lace ... so very far from
the real struggles that women have either with or without kids.
The idea that you would want to be part of this after spending your
twenties listening to grunge!! It's an insult to our generation's
experience.

Kim: 43, Single, UK/France

Just as there is a social taboo about talking about childlessness, there's also a taboo about telling the truth about motherhood. It's as if there's a cultural magic spell currently assigned to Motherhood with a capital 'M' and mothers aren't allowed to break it.

It's for this reason that I think it is worth taking the time to deconstruct how many of the 'meanings' we've assigned to motherhood actually make sense, and whether hanging on to these ideas is doing us any favours. It may be time to refresh these thoughts, as many of them are the products of the ideology of our times and not necessarily of our own thinking.

As Sammy Lee, a scientific consultant in one of London's top fertility clinics, wrote:

> As roles and rituals have been eroded, one of our last symbols of life are children. Children are a symbol of hope. So strong a symbol that children now dominate news media. We not only have a reborn fertility cult in the West, but also a cult of children, which has been a vital cog in the re-emergence of fertility itself as a modern cult.[56]

Ideology is that which everyone believes to be 'true', but it's actually a mixture of accepted prevalent beliefs that serve to support the dominant power group. Up until 500 years ago everyone thought the world was flat. That was an idea, not a truth, and around it was created a powerful ideology of Western Europe being at the centre of the world. So perhaps the 'belief' that a woman can only have a meaningful life if she is a mother may prove to be an ideological one and not the purely biological one that many of us have come to believe.

After all, there was a time when women dreamed of lives other than being mothers, precisely so that they could create lives of meaning.

It is the *meaning* we give to things, rather than the things themselves, that shapes our reality. And the meaning we give to things is something under our control, and can be changed.

How Our Childhood Colours Our
Feelings About Motherhood

What messages did you pick up about motherhood when you were a child? In my case, I was an unplanned baby born to a teenage mother and the sudden burdens and limitations of motherhood were a struggle for her. Having tasted the beginnings of freedom in the early 1960s, just a few years later she found herself 'respectably' and unhappily married, which was really the only choice for single mothers then unless you gave your baby up for adoption. And my mother made the incredibly brave decision not to.

Although I don't recall my mother ever telling me *not* to have children, she never actually encouraged me to have them either. Instead, she focused on all the amazing opportunities that awaited me as a child of the 1960s, with the movement for women's equality and the arrival of the Pill. One of the 'messages' that I absorbed from this was that motherhood definitely wasn't the only option for women. It wasn't hard to see that she longed to leave the narrow domestic world of motherhood and get back the freedom and independence she'd experienced as a teenager; I could tell that she keenly felt the bondage of her position as a dependent wife. So, another message I picked up from this was to 'have a career and don't rely on a man'. Also, growing up with an unhappy mother and an aggressive stepfather, I unconsciously came to associate childhood with fear and uncertainty, not love and safety. So, it was hardly surprising that I was in no rush to start a family of my own.

But it's not just a challenging childhood that may have left you with complex unconscious or unexamined beliefs about motherhood. For those of us who grew up in a 'perfect' family, the chances are it was perfect because your mother made it her life's work. And if you were an ambitious, bright girl, you might have looked at what her life entailed and thought, *I'm not sure I could ever sacrifice myself the way she did.* You could see that she worked her fingers to the bone on housework, gardening, baking, cleaning and worrying whilst seeming to have no life of her own outside that of being your mother. You could see that she got no obvious status or recognition for what she did: 'Oh, I'm just a housewife,' you may have heard her say, slightly apologetically. You may have never even heard people call her by her real name, but always as 'Mum' or 'so-and-so's mother'. Whilst she may have encouraged you to have a broader life for yourself, you may have been unconsciously aware of the difficulties of trying to combine those aspirations with the kind of full-time, hands-on mothering you experienced and absorbed as 'the right way to do it' . . .

> *Both my parents came from large families, and I am one of eight.*
> *My mother worked hard and never had much time for herself. I*
> *picked up a subliminal message that having kids, especially so*
> *many, was not all it was cracked up to be.*
>
> Tilda: 64, Married, New Zealand

It's not just our own family environment that will have given us ideas about motherhood; there's the broader social environment we grew up in and the religious and cultural beliefs we absorbed. At my school, our sex education classes consisted of one message: that getting pregnant was for losers and we'd be throwing away our lives. Looking back now, I can see that what our teachers were talking about were unplanned teenage pregnancies, but the message I took from it (and from talking to other women I have seen that I am not alone) is that the hard thing is *not* getting pregnant, and that having a child ruins your life. For those of us who went on to have infertility problems or to sometimes feel that *not* having a child has 'ruined our life' this rings pretty hollow.

Our current cultural fetishisation of motherhood was definitely not in place when I was a teenager, and the idea of our heroines getting pregnant and having babies was not something we wanted to know about or emulate. Debbie Harry having a baby? No way. (She never did, by the way.) Kate Bush having a baby? (She did, and disappeared from view, only recently resurfacing in the public eye.) It may not have been the same for everyone, but my peer group saw getting pregnant as a cop-out, uncool and somehow letting the side down.

However, I know other women who grew up during the same period whose families were more traditional and whose lives were focused around their faith and community. In order to go to university and have a career, these intelligent and ambitious young women had to go *against* their family's expectations that they would marry young and have children. Their mothers wept and did all they could to persuade them to 'settle down' instead. It was seen as an either/or choice, not a situation in which they could have both. In some ways those mothers were not as completely deluded as they seemed to us at the time. Sadly, it has certainly been the case for quite a few childless women that I've spoken with that the time spent on their education and career made it harder for them to find a partner in time to create a family. But still, none of them wished that they'd got married straight out of school and forgone their higher education.

If you were ambivalent about becoming a mother and hoped that 'life' would make that decision for you; that 'it would just happen one day', and then it didn't, it can be very painful to realise that some of that ambivalence came from your unexamined beliefs about childhood and motherhood. Finding this out too late is incredibly painful and can often compound the sense of being a failure as a woman because you didn't even manage to get clear on how you *really* felt about having a family – something which we hear is meant to be an 'obvious' and 'normal' desire for women. But 'normal' is a very loaded word, as human culture is far from 'normal', if it ever was. As I read on a fridge magnet, 'Normal is a setting on the dishwasher'! How can it be 'wrong' to get pregnant at sixteen but 'normal' to get pregnant in your thirties? We need to open our eyes to the cultural conditioning around us and see how we have taken on board such views, and ended up believing they're our own, even when they no longer serve us, and perhaps make us miserable.

Quite often I talk with women around the age of forty who've never wanted children and have been proudly childfree for a long time, but who are now wondering whether in fact they've made a mistake. They fear that maybe they do 'secretly' want a baby but that they just 'don't know it'. They fear waking up too late to their 'real' thoughts and feelings about having a family. So loaded and fraught has this seemingly 'obvious' and 'natural' decision become that there are now specialised 'Maybe Baby' coaches who work with women as they make this decision.

The fear of regret, of getting it wrong, seems to haunt many women as they come to the end of their fertility, because we now deem regret to be the shameful punishment for not making the right decisions. It seems that now most of us no longer fear that God will damn us, we fear damning ourselves. But there is no way to live a regret-free life, as far as I know, and it's important to remember that regret is an emotion that can be worked through and resolved, like all emotions. It's not a curse to be feared in the way that many of us seem to imagine. Regret may not be a 'nice' feeling, but hey, that's life. Having children often turns out not to be so 'nice' either . . .

Thinking that we are solely responsible for the outcome of our lives based on the quality of our own decisions can provoke an incredible level of anxiety. The philosopher Renata Salecl writes about this in her 2010 book, *Choice*, when she describes an experience many of us will identify with, that of going into a supermarket and being overwhelmed and paralysed by the anxiety of choice. Her personal nemesis proves to be a cheese shop in Manhattan where she finds herself getting angrier and more irrational as her options expand when all she wants is 'some cheese'.[57]

Choosing whether or not to be a mother is not one of those decisions you can take back to the shop, so the level of anxiety it can provoke can turn your life inside out if you don't realise what's going on. Because there is absolutely no way to future-proof the decision to become, or not become, a mother. You can weigh up the pros and cons for years, but ultimately, having a child is a leap of faith that you are committed to for the rest of your life. And if you get it wrong, you fear condemning yourself to a life of disabling regret. So, no pressure then!

EXERCISE 3
The Meanings of Motherhood

Grab a pile of Post-it notes or small pieces of paper (preferably in four different colours). Use them to write down individual words or phrases that come to mind in response to this exercise.

For each of the following prompts, write between five and ten responses on one colour of Post-it note. Then move on to the next prompt and the next colour. Don't think too hard about what you write. Just put the first things that come into your mind. It's not important at this stage that they make sense.

- Write one word or short phrase per note that springs to mind when you think of the word 'mother'. Repeat 5–10 times.

- Write one word or short phrase per note that springs to mind when you think of the word 'children'. Repeat 5–10 times.

- Write one word or short phrase per note about activities you like doing and that put you into a place of 'flow' (where time feels soft and passes in a flash). These might be activities that you feel are meaningful to you in some way, or they might not be. Repeat 5–10 times.

- Write one word or short phrase per note about ways of 'being' or 'feeling' that you enjoy (e.g. calm, loving, laughing ...). Repeat 5–10 times.

Arrange your responses in four vertical columns, with prompt 1 as the furthest left column, and prompt 4 as the last column on the right.
Now step back, and take a look.

- Can you begin to see that some of the things, states of being, ways of feeling, etc. (fourth column), that you have associated with motherhood and children (the first two columns) might actually be accessible through the activities you like doing (third column)?

• Can you see that some of the ways of being or feeling that bring you joy and meaning are actually open to you even *without* being a mother?

Choose one thing that you thought would only be accessible through motherhood (first and second columns) to do by carrying out an activity (third column) that brings meaning, joy or flow into your life (fourth column).

Commit to doing it this week. It doesn't have to be a big deal. If being in nature, sewing or writing feels meaningful and/or joyful to you, then do it. Often it's those things that have a 'creative' element to them that we resist the most. (We'll be looking more at why this might be in Chapter 10.)

There's no right or wrong way to do this exercise; it's just a way to start loosening some of the fixed associations in your mind that you can *only* be happy, content and live a life that has meaning for you if you are a mother.

Now, undoubtedly there are *some* aspects of being a mother that are irreplaceable – giving birth and the physical and emotional intimacy that passes between mother and child is not something we will ever experience. There are many things I will never experience in this lifetime, but that absolutely does not mean that I can't have a meaningful and fulfilling life without them.

Reflections on Chapter 4

In this chapter we've started to unpack some of the ideology surrounding motherhood in our culture and how we might have been influenced by it. Looking at this can be quite explosive, so if you have found yourself thinking, *I didn't buy this book so that she could run down motherhood!* I quite understand. When our cherished beliefs are challenged, our first reaction is often to shoot the messenger (and I didn't run down motherhood by the way!).

It can be galling to realise that we've invested so much of our life force chasing a 'fantasy' version of motherhood packaged by cultural conditioning and sold to us by the media. Even if we have sisters and friends with children and are privy to the day-to-day reality of their lives, those personal experiences still don't seem to counterbalance the vast weight of fantasy we are exposed to on a daily basis. Pronatalism is in the air we breathe; it takes a while to learn how to filter it out. Learning that this is not the case in every country, and that you don't face a barrage of celebrity bumps at the news-stand everywhere around the world, can bring on the first inklings that maybe what's going on around us is perhaps just a little bit nuts!

Reflecting on the messages we picked up in childhood can be a real eye-opener too and can bring up a lot of sadness and resentment. *If only I'd known this earlier* is not an uncommon thought and a really tough one to digest. When we are children, what we learn from our environment becomes part of our belief system of 'how the world is' and it becomes an unconscious template that we refer to throughout life, until we take the time to consciously unpack it. Although there is great freedom to be had in doing so, and then consciously choosing more helpful beliefs, it can also feel quite destabilising for a while. Often such new thoughts can radically change our view of ourselves, our choices and our lives, and it might all feel a bit overwhelming, and if there's part of you that wants to stick your fingers in your ears and say, 'La, la, la, not listening', I get it and if that's where you're at, that's absolutely fine. We can each only take on so much new information at a time. Take what you need from this chapter for now, and leave the rest. You can always revisit it later, if and when you feel you want to.

If you did the 'Meanings of Motherhood' exercise you may have been surprised, relieved or baffled by it, but I hope it has helped you to begin to question some of your fixed beliefs, namely that it is not true that all of the things you *believed* were denied to you forever because of not having children are *actually* denied to you. I hope it has also shown you that there *are* things you can start doing to feel better, although you may be surprised to find yourself digging in your heels and saying, 'No!' If you committed to an activity, you may have had to fight through a lot of resistance to actually do it. Strange as it may sound, our unhappiness may be an identity we've become used to. Beginning to let go of the identity of 'the crushed childless woman who will never be happy again' can be very provocative, and we may resist it fiercely. If you feel stubbornly resistant, that's good too. Stubbornness can be a form of anger, and anger is a very helpful energy when it comes to change ...

Change is never easy, even positive, hoped-for change. For now, whatever you've done or not done from this chapter, just know that by reading it you've already taken a big step and that your consciousness is shifting internally. The external changes will come when you feel ready. You can't force anyone else to change; and it's not that easy to force yourself to either. Time to try something different: kindness.

Grief is a
DIALOGUE,
not a
MONOLOGUE.

———

CHAPTER 4

Working Through the Grief of Childlessness

The Tunnel

Many of us will probably remember a time when thinking about motherhood was something that dominated our waking and sleeping thoughts – when it was literally all we could think about. On the very first blog I wrote for Gateway Women in April 2011, I described this state of mind as 'the tunnel':

> A narrow, cramped, claustrophobic space that gets more cramped as each year passes. Made for one. The only view ahead is a very narrow shaft of light, somewhere off in the distance. And behind you in the dark is every wrong decision, every failed relationship, every missed opportunity.
>
> The tunnel. A lonely, pressurised space where you can't turn round, can't reverse, can't go sideways. And your only guides in this fetid space? The polarised opinions of others and your own, by now, thoroughly freaked-out self. Because, even though you may or may not have given the issue much thought, you've suddenly realised with an awful sickening thud that if you don't have a baby, you're not a real woman, you've failed.[58]

The tunnel is a place where we lose touch with reality and ourselves as we become obsessed with the thought of having, or not having, a baby. It's what I've termed 'babymania'.

Some of us, myself included, can spend years in the tunnel, even decades. The experience is different for each of us but for me it was a sort of fugue state that I can only describe as a mixture of sleepwalking and panic. I lost some of the most precious years of my life whilst I was in the tunnel, made some terrible decisions and missed out on some fantastic opportunities. From talking to other women I know that my experience is something many of us can recognise, and which often only adds to our sense of shame.

> *I think it's probably the worst place to be – when there's that last bit of hope that you might become a mother, but it's dwindling each day. It is a truly horrible place to be. Slowly watching the death of your hopes and being powerless to prevent it. Reading about others in the Gateway Women community going through it, I can see how dreadful it is and I'm so glad that I have come through it. And crucially, I can now give myself compassion for what I experienced, because I can see other women also struggling, whereas before Gateway Women I thought I was 'being ridiculous' and 'over-emotional'.*
>
> Sophia: 50, Single, UK

The reason the tunnel can have *such* a destructive effect on our health, morale, personality, career, ambition and peace of mind is that it's actually another way to describe the first stage of grief: denial.

Grief is Good

In Western culture, we've become fairly hopeless at coping with grief, with loss. We fail to recognise its power, its meaning and its healing and run from it as if it were death itself. Yet grief is the emotional and psychological process that *enables* us to deal with loss. Avoiding it makes us emotionally stuck, unable to cope with life, unable to move forward.

Becoming aware of the possibility that we may not have children, that we may not have the family of our dreams, is a heartbreaking loss. Unlike many of the other losses we may have experienced, the end of fertility or the possibility of bearing a biological child is an irrevocable and definite loss. It's a kind of psychological death and it's profound. Facing up to it changes us forever.

What we, and others, often fail to realise is the depth and reach of our loss: that not only will we never have children, but we will never create our own family. We will never watch them grow up, never throw children's birthday parties, never take that 'first day at school' photo, never teach them to ride a bike. We'll never see them graduate, never see them possibly get married and have their own children. We'll never get a chance to heal the wounds of our own childhood by doing things differently with *our* children. We'll never be grandmothers and never give the gift of grandchildren to our parents. We'll never be the mother of our partner's children and hold that precious place in their heart. We'll never stand shoulder-to-shoulder with our siblings and watch our children play together. We'll never be part of the community of mothers, never be considered a 'real' woman. And when we die, there is no one to leave our stuff to, and no one to take our lifetime's learnings into the next generation.

If you take the time to think about it all in one go, which is more than most of us are ever likely to do because of the breathtaking amount of pain involved, it's a testament to our strength that we're still standing at all.

And yet, because the loss of our future children is an *invisible* loss, we often fail to recognise *ourselves* that what we are experiencing is grief, and others don't seem to have a clue what depth of pain and distress we are in. Some women are in such pain that they find themselves having suicidal fantasies. I did. It's not that I wanted to die, I just didn't want to live the rest of my life with this level of hurt.

If we miscarry, fail to conceive or never have the opportunity to try for a baby, our loss can remain invisible to others; it's known as 'disenfranchised grief' because it's grief that our society does not recognise and which consequently many of us feel shame for experiencing, if we allow ourselves to experience it at all.[59] And because our loss isn't recognised and reflected back to us with kindness and empathy we often give up seeking understanding from others and may instead learn to block out our pain with all kinds of self-medication, including drinking too much, overeating, overworking or becoming a sort of recluse. In doing so, we may remain stuck in a quagmire of unprocessed grief for years.

I actually first learned that what I was experiencing was acute grief while I was reading a sample of Jody's book online. For years I had had therapists ask, 'Well, have you grieved?' or say, 'You should take some time to grieve,' and I just could not access it, I could not express it because it was so vast. It took the breakdown of my adoption to let loose the floodgates; the grief was so powerful there was no way I could hide from it, stuff it down or contain it. This led to a near obsession with learning about grief, a growing understanding of it as a powerful natural healing process, and my now deep love, honour and respect for what I feel is the most neglected human condition.

Sally: 39, Married, Canada

If we had lost a living family by some tragic event, we would never expect ourselves to 'get over it'. Yet we, and others, expect those of us who are childless to pick ourselves up, dust ourselves off, count our blessings and get on with things. No wonder so many of us are struggling. The treatment we currently receive is not just neglectful, it's downright cruel. And sadly, knowing no better, many of us treat ourselves in exactly the same way.

I've come to understand grief as a form of love because it's created by love and it's a loving energy that heals us so that we can love life again. I like to imagine the moon, with its bright face towards us reflecting the sun, as 'love', and the dark side of the moon, in shadow, representing 'grief'. We need to go through the whole cycle in order for the sun to come out in our lives again. There's no other way round. We either stay in the dark or go through the dark and back out into the light again ...

Grief heals us, but we cannot do it alone. We cannot 'wait it out'. Time does not heal; grieving heals. But it cannot heal until it is witnessed and held jointly, with great tenderness, in the heart and soul of another. Just like love.

Just as one of the most painful romantic experiences is 'unrequited love', I think that disenfranchised grief is a form of 'unrequited grief' – a grief that is not allowed to be expressed, not allowed to be in a relationship. But grief cannot move into its active state, 'grieving', *without* a relationship because grief is a dialogue, not a monologue. And until we find a place to have that dialogue, either face to face, online or with a skilled therapist, it stays wedged in our hearts like a splinter. And it festers as it waits, infecting our life and our soul with sadness. It is vital that as childless women we give ourselves permission to grieve our losses and, in doing so, allow the grieving process to heal our hearts. Without grieving, we're stuck fast. And without empathetic company with whom to do our grief work, we can stay stuck for a very long time indeed. It's not as gloomy as it sounds because there's more to grief than sadness, and there's often as much laughter as tears. And those tears are healing ones. After all, not every culture is as nervous about grief as we are; in the Mayan tradition, grief is considered the highest form of praise, and crying as a form of prayer.[60]

Miracle Baby Stories

One of the ways that the culture colludes with us in our denial is with the 'miracle baby story'. This is the fairly predictable response we often get from others when the conversation strays into the fact that we don't have children, and never will.

The media features regular miracle baby stories of women who despaired for years about their childlessness and then had a baby after their nth round of IVF, through egg donation, surrogacy, etc. Or sensationalist stories of women in their fifties conceiving naturally, or women in their sixties and even seventies having babies using donor eggs. There is even a whole Wikipedia page[61] devoted to these extraordinary feats of human reproduction with data about the woman's age, father's sperm, reproductive technologies involved and live births resulting.

When someone says to us, 'But you mustn't give up hope! I read about this woman who ...' it's helpful to recall (and perhaps even to gently point out) that the reason these stories are in the media in the first place is because they are *news*. They are not the norm and they are referred to as 'miracles' because they are *rare*. Offering a childless woman this kind of 'hope' is akin to suggesting to someone with financial problems not to worry as they're going to win the lottery. And for every woman who makes the news or gets onto that Wikipedia page, how many other heartbreaking stories must there be of the women and couples who devastated their bodies, bank balances, relationships, careers and mental health chasing a miracle baby only to end up without one? Their stories are never told because they're not news, but they are just as much part of the story.

> *And those people that insist it is never too late – for what? To stop denying that you are middle-aged and no longer should be breeding? Or people who want to convince you that you must adopt or go to the sperm bank as a single woman – seriously? Drive myself to the maternity ward? Have a five-year-old to raise alone at the age of fifty-two? Get up at night and earn all the bacon? A kid at uni when I'm sixty-seven? C'mon!*
>
> Velda: 45, Single, South Africa

Just as *we* have difficulty accepting and processing our loss, so do others. As I've said, we've become culturally spooked by grief, by loss. It runs counter to the message of individualism, consumerism and science that *anything* can be fixed if you're smart enough, make good decisions, have enough data, think 'positively' and throw enough money at it.

Whether we realise it consciously or not, we humans, to a greater or lesser degree, feel each other's emotions – the mirror neurons in our brain fire when we see someone experiencing an emotion so that we feel the same. And so when others tell us about a miracle baby story, what they may be doing is using those stories as an unconscious shield to stop us feeling *our* pain so they can stop feeling what it triggers in them – *their* ungrieved losses. After all, we all carry so many. They may not realise what they are doing, but by defending themselves in that moment they deny us the very things we need to heal: understanding, recognition, empathy. Even just, 'I'm so sorry, that must be hard some days' would be a rare balm to our bruised souls.

Luckily, grief is patient, persistent and wise. It will keep seeking out that empathetic 'other' until your healing can be completed. Grief is not out to hurt you, it longs to heal you.

When I was forty-seven, a Gateway Woman posed a hypothetical question to me – she wondered what I would do if I were to meet a new partner and he wanted to try for a baby; would I be willing to go through IVF with a donor egg? This was not something I'd ever considered before.

'No,' I said, without hesitation.

'Wow, that seems pretty clear!' she said. 'How can you be so sure?'

I was pretty surprised myself but heard myself replying, 'Because I don't want to have a baby at this age. That time of my life has passed. I'm no longer looking to become a mother, that's over. I'm in a new phase of my life now. I've moved on.'

> *Grief had healed what was once a raw wound into a scar.*
> *And I can live with a scar, move forward with a scar. It*
> *will always be a tender spot, but it's no longer a wound.*

I will never 'get over' not having a family (it's not the flu), but that doesn't mean that I can't build a new life. There are moments when something touches the scar on my heart, and it can feel like all the air in my chest is suddenly gone. But these days I've learned that rather than contract against the pain, I literally open myself to it – pushing my shoulders back, imagining opening my chest area and heart, and I breathe in the pain, letting it flow through me and out of me. *More healing*, I say to myself, *another part of my heart healing*.

The things that trigger these moments are totally unpredictable. It can be the light bouncing off the shining hair of a child in the street as they turn their head, or a look that passes between a mother and her child. It can also be something that seemingly has nothing to do with children. For example, not that long ago a houseguest dropped a heavy saucepan onto my most precious set of china, a set of six plates that had been given to me as a wedding present by my maid of honour, my oldest friend from school. The plates had survived intact in storage for years after my divorce and had only just been unpacked. My guest was incredibly sorry and offered to replace the china, which I accepted, even though I knew that the set was a limited edition and irreplaceable – I couldn't bring myself to tell him that just yet. I walked away and went into the bathroom, feeling the loss keenly and wanting to wail with pain, yet also not wanting to upset him any further – after all, accidents happen. As I sat in the bathroom I thought of those plates, of the dear friend who had bought them for me, of meeting her when I moved to a new school at fifteen, of her sleeping in the bed next to me the night before my wedding. And then I thought, *What will happen to my china when I die? I've got no one to give it to.* It was an awful moment, but then I realised that once I was gone, they'd just be plates. Nothing more, just plates. I realised that it was all just 'stuff' and that what was important about them were my memories and *they* were still intact. I came out of the bathroom and told my guest not to worry about replacing them. 'They're just plates,' I said. 'Accidents happen.' In the past, something like that would have had me in bits for a week – the visceral realisation that I have no descendants, no one to whom anything of mine will mean anything. However, having done my grief work, such moments still hurt but, at a deeper level, I understand that I'm OK and that I can handle it. My reality no longer scares me, although sometimes, like on that occasion, it shocks me when I become aware of a new aspect of my loss.

Childlessness After Abortion

Although one in three women in the UK and USA[62] has had a termination by the age of forty-five, it's still a huge taboo to be open about this.[63] For those of us (myself included) who have gone on to remain childless after having had an abortion, there can be a dark shadow that hangs over us which says that somehow we're 'not allowed' to grieve our childlessness because we had an opportunity to be a mother and we didn't go through with it. It's another way of adding to the experience of disenfranchised grief, and a secret that even childless women rarely share with each other.

Looking back on my own experience, I was very young and absolutely terrified that having a baby was going to 'ruin my life'. It felt like the right thing to do at the time and, in hindsight, I can see that the twenty-year-old me wouldn't have made a very good mother; I still had a lot of healing from my childhood to do before that would be possible.

I didn't start grieving the loss of that child until the grief over my childlessness was well advanced, and it took me by surprise. I noticed that I was thinking about what might have been more often, and looking back at the young, confused, frightened young woman I had been with compassion and tenderness. I wanted to reach back to her and let her know that it's OK, it's all going to be OK. It was as if the part of me that will always be a mother was reaching out to 'mother' the lost and angry young woman I had once been.

Around about the same time I found myself in St Paul's Cathedral in London, supporting a group of Gateway Women who were attending a Saying Goodbye[64] memorial service for babies lost through unsuccessful IVF, miscarriage and stillbirth. At a certain point in the service, everyone was invited to come forward and light a candle, and to place them all together, each one a witness to a loss. Without any premeditation I decided that I needed to do the same for my baby too. For some reason I suddenly 'knew' he had been a boy, and so I named him 'Paul' after the cathedral, and took a lit candle for him to join all the others. I wept as I said a prayer for him and asked for his forgiveness. I thanked him for always being with me, and told him that I was sorry that I could not be his mother on this earth, although I was always his mother in my heart. I imagined the smoke from the hundreds of candles lifting his soul up and away from this complicated world, with all the other loved and missed children present in the cathedral at that moment. The tears I shed for him were perhaps the first tears I'd ever shed for my abortion, apart from tears of terror at the time. They were hot, healing tears and they opened a place in me that I didn't realise had been shut. I realised that through the loving power of grief, another piece of my heart had been healed.

> When I met my husband I was at the point where I had given up on the idea of marriage or having children. I'd had two abortions in my early and mid-twenties, both of them pretty traumatic emotionally, and I'd decided that I'd made my choices and had to live with them. But the shame never left me and it was something I didn't talk about anymore. Allowing my husband to truly love me was a challenge, and the shame became ever more present during this process. When we decided to try for a family I felt that my past would truly be behind me, that all that pain would have been worth it because I would eventually be able to have the baby I'd denied myself years ago. After three years of trying we were

told that I had unexplained infertility and I felt like it was my fault that our family would never be. The emotional rollercoaster took another turn, which led me to a place I wasn't prepared for: I couldn't tell anyone about my infertility diagnosis because I felt I didn't deserve their 'I'm sorry's', and that if they knew about my abortions, they'd say that I didn't deserve to be a mother. After all, that was how I felt inside. I began to find it hard to be around my friends and their children and I cried when I saw mothers with their babies – the pain was so great and I was so confused. A friend explained that I was grieving, which I found hard to accept because I felt I didn't deserve this grief.

Yasmin: 44, Married, UK

One of the hardest aspects of childlessness is that there are no rituals or ceremonies to mark the absence of the children we never conceived, never met, or only briefly. I realised with this service how powerful and necessary such rituals are, and how something physically lifted from me that day, and left me with a sweet space. Since then, I incorporate ritual as much as possible into my work with childless women, and I find it deeply creative and gratifying. I've included some ideas for rituals at the end of this chapter, and also at the end of Chapter 7.

Human beings of all cultures have ways of honouring thresholds from one part of life to another; it is vital that as childless women we do the same.

Coping with Other People's Joy

Whether we're coming to the end of our rope of hope, or know for sure that we're never going to be a mother, being around other people's joy at pregnancy and motherhood can really trigger our grief. It can also affect our sense of ourselves as 'nice' women if we find ourselves feeling envious and having dark and negative thoughts about someone else's 'good news'.

> *Announcements still sting and hurt, especially as they mostly now happen at work, where I don't feel able to explain things. I am fearing one of my team falling pregnant. We work very closely together and the thought of having to see her pregnancy at close quarters every day fills me with dread.*
>
> Natasha: 53, Single, UK

Jessica Hepburn, a veteran of nine unsuccessful IVF procedures and the author of *The Pursuit of Motherhood*, published in 2014, coined a brilliant word for the confusing combination of feelings that many of us will recognise around other women's pregnancies: 'melanjoy' – a combination of 'melancholy' and 'joy'.[65]

We each have to find our own way through such events and moments. Perhaps the hardest is the baby shower, something that has only recently become part of British tradition, but which has long been a fixture in other parts of the world. For some of us, avoidance of baby showers is the only way through, although it can be something our pregnant friends find hard to understand, and which may cast a shadow over that friendship. Others have found that a few years later, they've been able to reconnect with their friends and talk about why they couldn't attend.

> *I avoided baby showers for so many years that yes, the changes were quite drastic – I managed to create a world for myself where I no longer received these types of invitations or, if I did, they were very infrequent. The trade-off for the peace and decreased anxiety has of course been loneliness and knowing that I am missing out on some of life's most beautiful and joyful shared moments. But I had to put my own self-care first, and I don't regret not going, even while I wish it could have been different. Now that their children are a bit older and the 'baby fog' has lifted, I have approached*

*a few friends who I'd told excuses to, and let them know what
was my truth at the time; it has been an opportunity to heal and
deepen friendships that had faded over the years and I am very
grateful for their understanding and compassion. None of them
had hard feelings about it in any way so I think that's important to
know; emotions change over time for everyone, and this pain and
heartbreak will not always be so acute.*

Sally: 39, Married, Canada

For many of us who are still adjusting to the very real way that our
friends becoming mothers often means 'losing' them as friends, yet
another announcement can feel like a bell tolling on that friendship.
We've heard our friends say to us, 'It's not going to change anything,'
and we know that they mean it at the time, but they're probably going
to move towards a new circle of friends who are mothers, and that's
how it needs to be. And we're not mothers.

*Before, pregnancy announcements would affect me a lot. Now, less
so; I'm more used to them. But every time I hear one, I do feel like
one more woman has left my circle.*

Celeste: 39, Single, French Canada

Pregnancy announcements at work can be very hard when you're
grieving, and it does seem that it's become a much bigger deal than it
used to be. Social media has made it much easier to publicly announce
important life transitions than in the days before computers existed.
Perhaps the disparity between the current extreme social validation of
pregnant women and motherhood, and the disenfranchisement, silence
and shame around childlessness is thus particularly highlighted, and
we can feel both shut out *and* silenced.

Grieving Alone: Solo-Women's Grief

I experienced low-level anxiety throughout my twenties and thir-
ties, but it really hit me at forty-one, when I'd been through a lot
of stress at work and a former acquaintance emailed me that she'd
recently found the love of her life and they had married and had
a baby and she'd never been so happy. I wept all that day and my
grief was undeniable.

Sarah: 45, Single, USA

In a patriarchal society, our value as women is judged on our part-
nerhood and motherhood/grandmotherhood status. In my twenties
and thirties, I would have thought this was complete nonsense and,
as someone who considered herself a feminist, would have seen it as
rather backward-thinking. Imagine my shock when, as a newly divorced
woman of forty, I discovered how much 'status' my married state had
carried! Because I'd been in a relationship with my husband for sixteen
years, I'd come to take that status as something that belonged to 'me',
not to 'us' (well, to 'him' actually). I was baffled and hurt that, even
though our marriage broke down because of 'his' issues, and everyone
said I 'should have left him years ago', *he* was the one that was invited
to social events!

As I moved into my mid-forties and beyond my childbearing years
I became 'one of those childless women' (that's how I've heard myself
referred to) and then, as I settled into long-term singleness, I seem to
have become totally invisible to the world. No longer on any man's
sexual or mating radar, no one's wife, no one's mother; it's like I've
grown an invisibility cloak! Although I've come to terms with this and
now find my ability to be under the social radar quite liberating, it was
yet another aspect of my loss that I needed to grieve before I could find
even a scrap of a silver lining.

People don't get it − it's not just one generation's social activities
that you are not part of; it is all the generations that follow, and
all the activities that surround the whole school circle too. That's
how most adults relate outside of work − as someone's mother or
father. If you are not a mother, you just do not fit into the social
landscape very well, especially if it is family dominated in a mostly
suburban setting. It makes living arrangements and locations of
living very important for childless single people.

Velda: 45, Single, South Africa

Women who have children experience this too, a fading of their status and the beginning of invisibility as women as their fertility wanes, but the identity of 'mother' remains, as well as the status of being in a partnership if they are in a relationship. But those of us who have neither? We are the 'solos' or sometimes the 'double-whammies': single and without children. Double-whammy is a provocative label and it sits uncomfortably with me (and some other solo childless women too) because it feels victim-like, but there *is* an element of patriarchal victimisation involved, so perhaps the discomfort is to be acknowledged and brought into the open; it highlights a painful truth, that we are the butt of the patriarchal joke, the 'Old Maid' card in the antiquated (but still available) children's card game. Many women I've spoken to feel that other women judge them more harshly than men for being unpartnered and childless, but I think this points to a confusion between patriarchy as an ideology and patriarchy as a gendered point of view; both men and women have been conditioned this way, and in order to see things any *other* way requires some rigorous 'brainwashing' to clear the view. I feel that I've only cleared a small patch of glass in the foggy window of this conditioning and still have a long way to go.

Not having a life partner has been the most painful aspect of my
loss. I so wish I had a loving companion to share my life with.
Someone once said that 'Marriage is so that someone can witness

your life'. I've essentially witnessed my life on my own. That's only vaguely understood by others. Almost never discussed.

Libby: 68, Single, New Zealand/UK

'The Bitter Babe', a blog that ran from 2012–2014, had a strapline which I loved: 'Never married, over forty, a little bitter',[66] and it rang true with many women. Interestingly, my experience as a woman who *has* been married and who *did* try to have a child has a slightly higher 'status' on the social pecking order than that of a woman who has never been married or been in a long-term partnership in which she tried to get pregnant. You see, I get points for having been 'chosen' ... For double-whammies, the nasty unsaid comment that follows them around is, *What's wrong with her?* The answer, for all of the single, childless women I know, is this: absolutely nothing. And certainly nothing more than those women who have partners and are mothers. Sara Eckel debunks all of the 'reasons' brilliantly in her pithy 2014 book, *It's Not You: 27 (Wrong) Reasons You're Single*,[67] and if you haven't read it yet, you're in for a treat.

The grief of being solo and childless has its own flavour because *both* elements are disenfranchised and can be loaded with shame. And, like childlessness, sometimes it seems that all our friends and family can see when they look at a single woman is some kind of problem to be 'fixed'. And when they give up on that? Well, frankly we're often seen as the black ewe of the female line. Or that we're whinging about nothing because, didn't we realise, being single is 'fab', apparently! (Not that it isn't some days, but that's not the whole story.) Such comments as, 'Well, being in a relationship's not all it's cracked up to be, you know!' only serve to silence the single woman who absolutely *does know* that (she hasn't been living under a rock), but who'd still like the chance to have her own relationship, ups and downs and all! It's like saying to a childless woman, 'Kids are more trouble than they're worth!' and wondering why the woman in front of you has gone a strange colour and suddenly needs some fresh air ...

Grieving Together: Navigating Grief
as a Couple

Whether you are childless as a couple due to infertility, because your partner doesn't want children, doesn't want more children or for any other reason, navigating the grief process as part of a couple also presents its own challenges. For those who are single, the pain of experiencing it alone is acute; for those in a partnership, often it is the sense of 'separateness' within the relationship during grief that cuts deep.

> *One of my biggest challenges was the feeling of being utterly and completely alone within my marriage. After receiving a diagnosis of infertility I went through a period of shame and anger that felt very black and deep to me. It was one of the hardest, darkest periods that I faced through this whole fifteen-year journey. At that time my husband – himself dealing with his own feelings about my diagnosis and what that meant for us – was at a loss as to how to reach or help or support me. From my perspective at the time, I felt completely abandoned by him, let down and very angry that he was giving so much attention to his work at a time when I needed him more than I ever have.*
>
> Hannah: 47, Married, UK

If we think of grief as a form of love, we might realise that it will therefore be a unique and subjective experience for each of us, as love is. For couples who share love, it can be terrifying how differently they experience the grieving process, as it feels like it's threatening the foundations of their love for each other, and brings up the fear that perhaps the relationship will be yet another collateral loss of childlessness.

For men in our culture, conditioned to believe that being strong and not showing emotion is 'manly', finding a way to express their grief can be challenging. Robin Hadley, a British academic who has been researching and writing about male childlessness for some time, believes that men and women have the same 'deep grief' over childlessness but that 'we are socialised to express bereavement behaviour along gendered dogma lines.'[68] In other words, big boys don't cry ...

> *It was hard because I didn't know how to help my wife; I felt there was nothing I could do to help her with her pain. Grief showed up for me by shutting me down a little, I guess, and I didn't really realise I was grieving probably. I just thought that I was fine all the time, and I had to be strong or whatever for my wife, and later on I realised I was actually pretty messed up. There was quite a long time where I didn't go out and do anything. So I started mountain biking and that helped me deal with my grief, and it got me out and I started to feel better.*
>
> John: 42, Married, Canada

Sexual intimacy can take a real hit from childlessness too, particularly, but not only, for those who have experienced unsuccessful infertility treatments. The invasiveness of the procedures, and the resulting trauma, can knock a woman's sense of her body as a site of joy and pleasure completely out of sight. Indeed, recent research has shown that as many as 50 per cent of women who had undergone fertility treatments had symptoms of post-traumatic stress disorder (PTSD), as compared to the 8 per cent of the general population who are thought to suffer from it.[69] And even without PTSD, trying to rebuild sexual intimacy once you know that children aren't part of the picture is hard, let alone when you're grieving and experiencing physical difficulties such as erectile dysfunction and loss of libido, which are common during and after infertility.[70]

And so intimacy itself, and the comfort it used to bring, can become something else to grieve, compounding the loss. Some couples turn away from sexual intimacy in the relationship at this point, and it's not hard to understand why. However, perhaps knowing that it's part of the grieving process rather than necessarily pointing to a deep rift in your relationship may help to get you through and back in touch with each other joyfully when you're both ready. Indeed, a ten-year follow-up research project of couples who were childless after IVF showed that infertile couples have a lower divorce rate and that 'contrary to expect-ation, infertility does not always have a negative impact on marital cohesiveness and satisfaction'.[71]

> *In the beginning it made me very sad that everything my body had gone through during puberty and all of the years of menstrual cycles were for naught. Now I'm realising that we are lucky that we can have sex whenever we want, with the bedroom door wide open, no kids to worry about.*
>
> Kyla: 43, Married, USA

Something I've noticed frequently in my work with partnered child-less women is that it is often as a woman comes out of the worst of her grief that her partner seems to be able to grieve more. I'm not aware if this is the same with lesbian partners (who are mostly neglected in discussions about childlessness), but in heterosexual couples, I do wonder if some of the masculine conditioning around 'being strong' is at work? It often comes as a great surprise to the women I work with to discover the depth of feeling their partner had harboured all along, and many of them wished they'd seen evidence of it earlier, as they would have felt less alone in their grief.

> *My partner has been very supportive and the more I have opened up the more able he has been to support me. I have learned, though, that it is OK for us not to be in the same stage of grief and that when this happens we may not be able to give each other everything that we need. For example, as I came out of the worst of my grief I noticed that he went into his grief more deeply – maybe because he gave himself permission to feel it more deeply now that I need less support. My partner tends to internalise his grief more, whereas I need to talk (and talk!),*

and being able to catch those times when he wants to talk can
be tricky.

Heather: 40, Married, UK

For some couples, seeking outside support from an infertility counsellor can be a great help. Often, infertility clinics do offer a 'follow-up'
counselling session, but it's usually much too soon to be of use as it
comes hot on the heels of a decision to stop treatment and the shock
that comes with that. Whether infertility was part of your story or
not, if you and your partner are struggling to come to terms with
your childlessness, do consider going to see an infertility counsellor,
as they understand the grief of childlessness. However, if you have
had treatment, you might prefer to see one not connected to any
clinic, so that you don't risk being triggered by such environments or
associations.

Backed-up Grief

For many of us, the experience of moving into grief may bring up other
ungrieved losses. It's as if our unconscious says, 'Right, she's finally
grieving! Let's get all this other stuff that's been lying around here up
and out while we can!' This can feel pretty overwhelming and scary and
the stuff that can surface in our body, heart and mind can feel quite
shocking: *Why I am thinking about* that *again?*

> *I think in the beginning of my grief work one of the ungrieved losses*
> *that came up for me was how lonely and frightened I was as a little*
> *girl because my mother spent so much time away from me in hospital.*
> *I had truly underestimated the impact of that on my childhood.*

Laura: 47, Single, UK

For me, the loss of my marriage and my ex-husband's decline into
the depths of alcoholism and addiction (I expected to hear of his death

daily), losing our cherished home and the interior design business we'd run together for a decade, the onset of menopause and my childlessness all came in the same few terrible years. And yet there was still space for my grief to throw up the little soul I'd aborted, the boyfriend I'd had before my husband who I remained close to and who died young of a brain tumour, and the grief of losing the major part of my peer group.

> *I realised that I had never truly grieved for the loss of my father,*
> *for the loss of my childhood, for the loss of my true self, for the lost*
> *years ... When my beloved cat died three years ago, I grieved in*
> *a way that I had never done before and all my losses rose up and*
> *overwhelmed me. I've worked through much of the grief now by*
> *recognising and acknowledging that my grief was very real and*
> *that ignoring it was preventing me from healing.*
>
> Marianne: 63, Married, UK

The loss of a pet triggering a much bigger wave of losses is quite common in the experience of women I've worked with, and can be really frightening. For me, before I understood that the implosion of overwhelming feelings I was experiencing was grief, I seriously wondered if I was going mad. One of the things I've learned about grief is that in most cases it has its own sort of 'gauge' as to how much you can deal with and, although it might feel like it's too much, once we reach our 'maximum', the wave begins to recede very soon after. Quite often, periods of intense grief (a big wave) are followed by a more pleasant time paddling about in the shallows, looking in rock pools and thinking, *Oh, I feel so much better, I must be through my grieving.* And then, a few days, weeks or months later, another wave crashes over you. But hopefully by then you'll have built up your resources by doing your grief work, and after you've been through the cycle a few times, you might even get better at noticing the wave building on the horizon and feel more prepared for it ...

I think grief was rather the other way around for me. My child-
lessness grief was suppressed until other losses were grieved – the
loss of a long-term partner due to unfaithfulness, the loss of a life
in another country that I thought I would be living and was happy
in, the loss of my house, the loss of all that I thought was true and
real in my life at that time. It was only after I had dealt with how
that was for me in terms of grief that the childlessness reared up
and bashed me good and proper between the eyeballs. It was a
shocking and life-changing moment.

Claude: 44, Single, UK

When grief doesn't come in waves but rather feels more like you are stuck underwater, it may have become what is known as 'complicated grief', which is more serious and requires that you seek professional support. The Center for Complicated Grief describes it as something that 'complicates' the natural 'wound healing' of grief.[72]

The most difficult aspect of my grief and loss has been the many,
many layers, and figuring out that each of them requires its own
attention and its own process. It is so painful, the first year I was
numb and the second and third years were excruciating. This
is something I wish I'd been taught (in school, in life) about the
intensity of the pain, the debilitating all-over physical, emotional,
mental and spiritual agony, that it is bearable with adequate
support, and that most importantly we do not, and should not,
have to suffer through it alone.

Sally: 39, Married, Canada

About 7 per cent of adults who've experienced the loss of someone they consider important experience complicated grief. A lack of under-standing around you, hostile treatment from others and a history of anxiety and depression, among other factors, can make it more likely.[73] I imagine it like a grief wave that doesn't recede to give you breathing space. Some clues that your grief may be stuck might be that you're barely able to take care of yourself (eating, sleeping, washing, dressing), you can't think about anything else except the loss of the family you longed for, you've pretty well cut off all contact with the outside world and you may feel that life's not worth living anymore. You may even have started to formulate a plan to end your life. This level of distress, which any of us grieving childlessness may have periods of, is intolerable to the psyche if we get stuck in it. At this point, it's really important to seek help; even dialling the emergency services would be fine, whatever time it is. Or you might feel more comfortable with the anonymity of a telephone helpline such as the Samaritans in the UK or any type of suicide hotline, which you can call even if you're not feeling suicidal because the people working for these services will be sympathetic to the level of distress you're in and will take it seriously. You may prefer to book an appointment to see a grief or bereavement counsellor. Whatever you do, do something and do it right away. With support, complicated grief can resolve back into regular grief, and you can resume your recovery journey into the next part of your life. Please don't try to tough this out. Your suffering isn't some kind of cross you have to bear, and whatever dark thoughts you may be having, you don't 'deserve' to feel this terrible.

Grandchildren Grief

First the good news: fully grieving not becoming a mother will hopefully mean that when your peers start having grandchildren, it won't be as hard as you might fear. It's not that there won't be griefy moments sometimes – because healed grief leaves a scar, and a scar will always be a tender spot.

However, if by the time other people's grandchildren start appearing you *haven't* fully grieved motherhood, but have instead perhaps found a way to push your pain aside and move on as best you could, you may find that you are unexpectedly thrown back into despair. Not having grandchildren may bring back the pain of not having been a mother, and friends that you may have reconnected with once their children had left home once again start becoming less available.

> *I have finally accepted my childlessness. Goodness, it seems semi-miraculous to be able to state that, but I do fear the next stage when my friends start to become grandparents.*
>
> Natasha: 53, Single, UK

I had a hint of what's to come during the depths of my grief when my then teenage goddaughter walked up to me with a mutual friend's baby on her hip and said, 'I can't wait till I have my own baby!' With a sickening lurch I realised, *It's all going to happen again one day – watching everyone but me become grandparents.* The vision of this beautiful young woman at the very beginning of her childbearing years was so archetypal, so full of promise and joy, and yet so coloured by my own loss. A bittersweet tear popped out of the corner of my eye and joined my genuine delight in her excitement, as well as my fervent hope that *her* dreams of a family come true. *May she never know the taste of these tears, I prayed.*

Many older childless women have told me how painfully left out they feel because of not having grandchildren. For many of them there was little opportunity to grieve the loss of motherhood at the time; coming from a more buttoned-up era emotionally, they tell me that they were told to just 'get on with things'. However, as other people's grandchildren come into view, the feelings of grief and despair that may surface can take them aback.

Think about it for a moment: how many empowering and happy images can you find in the media of women or couples over the age of sixty that don't include grandchildren somewhere in the picture?

Although it may not feel like it's got anything going for it, the pain that comes up around grandchildren is actually grief signalling to you that you have another opportunity to heal the pain of not becoming a mother. And by addressing this loss, as well as that of your grandchildren, you'll find yourself much more able to live the next act of your life as a powerful, happy and integrated older woman.

> *Now I am very happy for my friends and share with them their joy in their grandchildren. I think that is because they are women with many dimensions and interests, and not solely identified with their status of mother and grandmother. In any social situation when I am with women of my generation who talk incessantly about their grandkids and compete with one another over whose grandchild is the most special or intelligent or gifted, etc., sometimes I change the subject, but I notice it doesn't take long for the default setting to kick in again. I become bored and move away to talk to someone more interesting.*
>
> Tilda: 64, Married, New Zealand

Healing your grandchildren grief will enable you to celebrate the life you've got and enjoy your friends' stories of their grandchildren without losing the plot. Well, that's the plan anyway. I'm afraid there's nothing that'll inoculate you against boredom or irritation!

A Guide to Grief: the Five Stages of Grief Model

The Five Stages of Grief model was developed by Elisabeth Kübler-Ross as a hypothesis from her work with terminally ill patients and was set out in her 1969 book *On Death and Dying*.[74] Although it has often been contested, it has not been bettered and has been hugely influential in the West in helping us to understand the power, process and necessity of grief in dealing with loss.

Sometimes, Kübler-Ross's model is referred to as DABDA, which is an acronym for the names of the five stages:

1. **D**enial

2. **A**nger

3. **B**argaining

4. **D**epression

5. **A**cceptance

The linear, list-like nature of Kübler-Ross's model can give the impression that grief is a tidy process, one that moves cleanly and clearly from one stage to the next, but there are many who prefer to visualise it as something slightly more organic: as a spiral. Kübler-Ross recognised this herself, commenting later that, 'the stages are not linear. People do not necessarily go through all of them.'[75]

A spiral has a trajectory, but one which curves and dips back on itself, as does grief. I also think that different parts of our experience are in different positions on the spiral – we are not completely in denial about everything related to our loss, and whilst we might be aware of the fact that we will never have a child, we can still be thrown back into depression or anger by the realisation that we will never have grandchildren.

Grief is a powerful, life-changing human emotional process, like love. Indeed, another Elizabeth, Queen Elizabeth II, said that 'grief is the price we pay for love'.[76] But I have a different view.

I have come to believe that grief is actually the <u>gift</u> of love. We cannot grieve that which we have not loved; and we cannot be healed from the loss of that love without grief.

Grief is not about getting over a loss, but about healing around it until that loss is integrated into our new identity. The tears of grief are not a sign of weakness but of healing.

So, whilst the Kübler-Ross model gives us a framework to understand grief and a shared language to use as we support each other in our grief work, we need to realise that grief remains an experience as subjective for each of us as love is.

If we think of grief as a form of love, rather than a set of steps to arrive at a destination, it becomes easier to understand that it is ever changing, often surprising, deeply revealing and not always convenient. Transformation is never straightforward.

Denial: the First of the Five Stages of Grief

We can only be aware of those things that we are no longer in denial about or which we are in the process of coming out of denial about. There will always be some things we are *still* in denial about; it's part of being human. In *The Language of Letting Go*, Melody Beattie describes denial as a duvet that we pull over our heads to protect us from a painful awareness and which gradually, as the conditions around us feel safer, we pull down, bit by bit.[77] I like the gentleness of picturing it as warm and cosy protection, rather than something we're doing wrong by avoiding thinking about it.

There's nothing wrong with denial, despite the way it's bandied about in popular parlance; it's a very wise psychological mechanism that protects us from anguish we're not yet ready to deal with.

Without denial to protect us, if we were to feel the full force of our losses in one go, rather than gradually, the shock might well be unendurable.

Perhaps continuing with infertility treatments long after we could afford to, either financially or emotionally, is a form of denial. Or being unshakably convinced that we would have one of those 'miracle babies' – after all, that's what everyone keeps telling us. It may be as simple as chopping a few years off our age, or as complex as allowing someone to presume that a niece or nephew is our own child without correcting their mistake.

You might realise that when you used to convince yourself that having periods meant you were still fertile you were in denial about the quality of your remaining eggs. Or perhaps you used to scour the media for any stories about women your age having children and keep those articles like talismans. Or then again, perhaps you let people think you were still trying to have a baby long after you and your partner had stopped fertility treatments.

In twelve-step recovery programmes (like Alcoholics Anonymous), denial is often explained by the acronym **D**on't **E**ven k**N**ow **I A**m **L**ying. There is a lot of truth in this (no pun intended!) because denial is impervious to logic or reality. It protects us completely. You might even recall that before you fully acknowledged that you were never going to become a mother someone tried to discuss it with you, perhaps even to offer you some support, and you brushed them off slightly aggressively as having got your situation 'completely wrong'. That's denial.

Anger: the Second of the Five Stages of Grief

When we resent the fact that 'she' got a family but we didn't. When we find ourselves saying unkind things about 'mothers'. When we feel bitter, judgemental and outraged by the way we are treated by society as childless women, what we're experiencing is anger.

There's nothing wrong with anger, despite its bad reputation. Like all human emotions, it's there for a reason – it's a response to injustice. It's a protection mechanism.

However, we need to be wise in understanding the difference between healthy anger and unhealthy anger. Healthy anger is a motivating force that gives us the energy to make changes in our life. Unhealthy anger shows up as resentfulness or bitterness and a negativity that may form a shield that keeps everyone at a safe distance. I've met childless women so angry that it's very hard to be in their presence at all ...

Some of the anger we feel about how overlooked we are as women because we don't have children is what I would think of as justified anger. It encourages us to change the way things are. It doesn't give us the right to berate anyone, but it does give us the nerve to stand up for ourselves and for others who are not yet ready to do so.

Bitterness and spiteful remarks may be signs that we are stuck in grief-related anger about our childlessness. Those feelings *will* pass as we move through our grief, but they can reappear when we come face to face with a new version of an old situation – like an ex-partner having a baby or grandchild, or even just a TV advert showing a multi-generational family including children and grandchildren.

Anger is a very potent feeling to experience, both emotionally and physically. It stimulates our fight-flight-freeze response and fills our system with powerful chemicals that can result in stress-related illness and erratic behaviour if not dispersed through physical activity or an emotional release of some kind. Whilst punching a pillow doesn't work for everyone, going for a run or (one of my favourites) deep-cleaning the bathroom, can really help to disperse the biochemicals produced as part of the anger response. Some kind of creative practice like painting, singing or gardening can be a helpful release too – I find writing to try and correct or respond to injustice allows me some resolution. After all, that's how Gateway Women began.

Anger doesn't always look or sound angry. Some women, brought up in families and cultures where girls weren't 'allowed' to be angry, turn it on themselves instead and overeat, drink and develop a super-critical inner voice that makes everything they do 'wrong'. An inner bitch can be as vicious, if not more so, as an outer one. (More on taming your Inner Bitch in Chapter 9.)

Alternatively, some of us may have learned whilst very young how to use anger as a way to suppress or hide our vulnerability and know just how to use it to protect ourselves. In this case, grief may turn our anger dial right up to 10 and we may be furious with absolutely every-one and everything. White-hot fury at the world is understandable, but it's a scorched-earth policy and you may lose jobs, partners, friends and the support of your family if you don't realise soon enough that it is burning up your life. Anger management classes aren't going to help; you need to do your grief work.

Anger can show up in all kinds of ways: the 'flight' response may show up with you running a marathon or single-handedly landscaping the garden. It makes things happen, so you may change careers, leave your partner and move country whilst under its galvanising influence, only to wake up one day and wonder what the hell happened. The 'fight' response often manifests in argumentative, unreasonable, fault-finding intolerance towards yourself and others and destructive behaviour. And the 'freeze' response (playing dead in mammals) can include emotional paralysis, staying in an unhealthy relationship, an inability to make decisions and a loss of libido, but may also show up in withdrawal behaviours such as substance abuse, overwork or obsessive TV or internet use – anything that 'zones us out'.

Despite all this, and although we may not realise it, anger is a loyal friend. It may not be nice or pretty, but it's a hell of an activating emotion. Anger is the fire of life, the fire in the belly. It makes stuff happen if you let it. Using it wisely can take a lifetime; suppressing it is an illusion – it just goes underground and it will come up somewhere else.

Bargaining: the Third of the Five Stages of Grief

Bargaining is a strange state and a hard one to pin down sometimes. It involves negotiating with reality, or 'magical thinking' as a way of trying to make our loss go away.

Whilst there is still hope of having a baby, bargaining tends to take the form of things we could change in order to make it more likely that we will have a child. It might be that we think that if we're 'a better person' we'll get pregnant, or we think of ways we could behave that might make us 'deserve' to win the lottery and be able to afford to have a baby on our own or pay for more fertility treatments. We might return to a faith of our youth or develop obsessions or superstitions.

However, once we are *sure* that we are no longer able to have a biological child, bargaining takes more subtle forms. We might decide that if we stop this or start that we'll meet a partner with children. It's also not uncommon to fantasise about friends or siblings being killed suddenly so that we become guardians of their children. These thoughts are normal, even though they shock us with their ghoulishness.

We may also enter a phase of compulsively counting our blessings as a way of warding off our grief over childlessness, trying to trick ourselves into thinking that it's a good job we didn't have children. We might find ourselves reading the newspapers specifically to see how many terrible things are happening in the world that *our* children aren't going to have to experience. Or we might focus on the negative aspects of our personality or circumstances and decide that it was probably for the best that we didn't inflict these on our children. And then, when something unforeseen and difficult happens, like a relationship breakdown, job loss or chronic illness, we might hear ourselves saying, 'Thank goodness I didn't have a child!'

Alternatively, we may focus slightly obsessively on the positive aspects of our unchosen freedom from the responsibility of childrearing, perhaps by going on wild spending sprees, booking exotic and adventurous holidays and telling ourselves, 'I couldn't have afforded this if I'd had children!' We may find ourselves seeking out non-child-friendly activities and even taking up high-risk sports or hobbies because we think that no one's ever going to rely on us to be 'the responsible one'. We might decide to spend our life-savings *now*, because who do we have to save it for?

We may even try to convince ourselves that we didn't *really* want children, but rather that we were just going along with social conventions, with what was expected of us. And I'm not saying there might not be some truth in that ...

What's happening is that we're trying to weigh our loss against life and decide that it's OK. But it's not. If it were, it wouldn't be the first thing that sprang to mind when our life took a new turn.

It's as if we are still holding a space in our life for that child. We aren't letting go, not completely, not yet.

We may even fantasise about some kind of Faustian pact whereby we make a sacrificial deal with a higher power in order for the chance to become a mother. It's not logical, but it's the way we work through all the possible – and impossible – ways we might try to avoid the pain of our loss before we are ready to face and accept it.

Depression: the Fourth of the Five Stages of Grief

Withdrawing from the world to lick our wounds is a natural part of adjusting to loss. It's the time when we give up hope and face what's underneath all our denial, anger and bargaining – the reality of what we've lost: the loss itself.

Being depressed is not necessarily always a problem; it has a valuable part to play in giving us the rest and space we need to reconstruct our identity after losing someone or something very dear to us. It's a natural response. However, when it moves from a deep sadness into a clinical depression that does not lift, it's important to see a doctor. One of the symptoms of clinical depression can be that you don't realise you're depressed, so if others close to you suggest that you are and yet you hadn't thought so, it might be a good idea to get it checked out.

The depression that is a part of grief will pass when it has given you the space, rest and introspection you need to move forward with your healing journey.

A typical thought I've heard from many women in the depression stage of the grief cycle is, 'What's the point of anything anymore? I'm never going to be a mother.' Such thoughts, and trying to find a way to resolve them, can form cyclical and repetitive patterns of thinking that go literally round and round until we are mentally exhausted. In fact, depression used to be called 'mental exhaustion'.

Sometimes, we may withdraw from our partner and from sexual

intimacy because it seems pointless if there is no hope of a baby. We may push our partners away, trying to make them leave us because we have 'failed' them. We might stop taking care of ourselves, not being bothered to make an effort with the way we look, or to stay fit. We may feel de-sexed as women now that we will never be 'real women'. We may wonder what the point of us is as women if we are never to be mothers.

There may also be fear and anxiety in the depression stage as we begin to contemplate the rest of our lives without children, of growing old and dying without them to care for us. We may fear that our partner will leave us, or that we will never meet someone and will be alone and miserable for the rest of our lives. (We'll be looking at ways to think differently about these fears in Chapter 12.)

We may cry and mourn in the stereotypical sense, perhaps feeling regretful and unable to see, engage with, or in some cases even *look* at children because our pain is so acute. We may find that it seems we are suddenly surrounded by children, by pregnant women, by grand-children, and that withdrawing from the world seems to be the only way to cope. We have no energy, our sleep patterns change (insomnia or sleeping much more than usual) and our appetite changes too (usually a loss of appetite, but sometimes eating a lot of comfort food).

We reject those who try to cheer us up and can be quite aggressive towards them if they persist; we are in a deeper place than that, and we know that's where we need to be.

Acceptance: the Fifth of the Five Stages of Grief

Ah, acceptance. Sounds nice, doesn't it?

In reality, it's a mixed bag. Because what it means is accepting fully and completely right down to our very bones that we will never have children, never be a mother, never be a grandmother. That the millions of years of genetic feats of survival that created us stop here. That when we die, we die more absolutely than someone who knows that they 'live on' in their children.

> **Acceptance is about coming to terms with our destiny
> and making peace with it. It doesn't mean we like it, or
> that we think it's fair. It just is what it is.**

It doesn't mean that we won't be sad about how things have worked out, but rather that we are no longer hopeful of any other outcome and so we stop fighting it. We accept it.

Acceptance does not mean that we go quietly. But what it *does* mean is that the energy that was locked up in our grief becomes available to us again, to dedicate towards a new future. Our past, and all the wrong turns, twists of fate, decisions made when five years old and left unexamined, biological complications, timing misses and misunderstandings that led to our childlessness become less important. We stop raking over them, we forgive ourselves and others involved in the drama, and we move on. We start thinking about what's next, rather than what might have been.

Grief heals. What was once an open wound is now a scar. And we are ready to face life again, on its terms, not ours. We are ready to start thinking about our Plan B.

How Long Does Grieving Childlessness Take?

Grieving our childlessness, as you may already know and which I hope I've illustrated in this chapter, is a complicated business. Our grief doesn't come in a tidy drawer labelled 'childlessness', but is diffuse, messy and multi-layered. Aspects of it can surface to be worked on at any point in our life. I consider myself to be 'in recovery' from childlessness rather than 'over it' and it's something that will be a part of me for the rest of my life. I have grown around and through this loss, but I haven't 'got rid of it'. And, several years into my recovery, nor would I want to – it's part of my story, an integral part of who I am.

When women ask me how long grieving is going to take, I imagine that what they are asking is, 'How long am I going to feel *this* bad?', and I think that although it varies from woman to woman, it really depends on how much grief work you feel able to do. However, with dialogue of some kind, I've seen women feel a good deal better in one year, and much better again a year after that. When you consider the depth of pain and confusion, this is really rather quick, although a lot of women are appalled: 'That long?!' they say, 'I'm going to feel this bad for two years?' And again, the answer is both yes and no. Because there will be days, maybe even today, reading this book, when you feel a lot better, and days, perhaps tomorrow, when you feel pain and sadness. But once we begin our grief work, things can begin to shift quite quickly, and you can start moving forward with life again. You're not going to feel 'this bad' all the time for the whole of the next few years ... there will be some days that are easier than others, and some days that are fantastic.

Research released in 2015 from the UK charity, Sue Ryder, found that:

> People grieve on average for two years, one month and four days after losing a loved one, but talking through emotions can help people feel better sooner [...] people who did not have any support grieved for an additional eight months, three weeks and five days on average.[78]

These figures focus on an accepted form of grief: losing a living loved one, as opposed to the disenfranchised grief of childlessness. I was interested to find out that two to three years seems to be the average, but this is for the active process of 'grieving' rather than being 'in grief', and in my experience you can still be in grief for your child-lessness decades later if you haven't had some support to process your grief. Aspects of the loss can resurface at any time, even after you're through the first couple of years, although with conscious grief work and tools, the 'griefy' moments become less severe, pass more quickly and are more infrequent. The waves subside, but the tides continue ...

Grief is passive; grieving is active. The good news is that once you begin your grief work you'll find that grief *isn't* a life sentence of misery, but that it can start 'moving' quite quickly. This can also be slightly bewildering and may bring up feelings of guilt. I used to get pangs of guilt when I was newly in recovery from my childlessness, thinking things like, *Well, if I've managed to get past my grief, that probably means I didn't really want to be a mother*. Even at the time, I knew that it wasn't 'true' because I knew how badly I'd suffered, and how much I'd lost during those years of longing before I arrived at acceptance. In time, I came to understand that these thoughts were perhaps the childless version of 'survivor's guilt' and were a further (illogical) part of processing my experience as I came to have faith that I really was OK, that I really had made it through the worst experience of my life. I think part of me expected my grief to come back and bite me if I didn't keep an eye on it! It took me a couple of years of continuing to feel better before I felt totally confident that it wasn't a 'blip' of some kind and that I really was whole again.

Grieving is an organic process, not a linear one, which can be very hard to accept in our predominately mechanistic, left-brained, analytically oriented culture. It may seem like an illogical process when you're in it, because it is – it's an emotional, psychological and physiological process that's rewiring you from the inside out. And that takes a bit of time and can be a bit of a bumpy ride!

Doing Your Grief Work

What is grief work? Grief work is simply finding a way to process your grief with others who totally 'get it'.

Suggestions for Rituals and Ceremonies

Some of the earliest human rituals we have knowledge of are connected with burial rites. The need to acknowledge loss is a very deep part of what it is to be human. For those of us dealing with disenfranchised grief, a ritual or ceremony can be a powerful way to mark our loss and can be a huge help in moving us towards acceptance. Organisations and resources that you may wish to explore to support you with this are listed in the Appendix. However, here are a few easy-to-organise rituals that I and other Gateway Women have found both moving and helpful:

- Create a 'memorial garden' somewhere in your garden to honour your loss. You might like to plant something special there and have a ceremony for the planting, and perhaps bury a significant object so that the roots of the new life will wrap around your sorrow and hold it tight. If you have any photos or memorabilia that you feel it's time to let go of, you can burn them and mix the ashes in with the earth.

- Create a ritual 'shrine' for your longed-for family somewhere private in your home. You might include flowers, candles, any objects that you associate with your loss (such as embryo photos, sonograms, letters), perhaps any baby clothes or toys that you were saving from your own babyhood or had bought or borrowed in preparation for motherhood. The idea is to create a place you can visit and sit and be with your grief and honour it.

- Do the 'Decluttering Your Dreams' exercise at the end of Chapter 7.

- Attend or organise a memorial service for childlessness either within your own faith community or in a secular/non-denominational environment. It can be very powerful to hold the ceremony outdoors, too.[79]

Further Suggestions for Grief Work

Here are some other ideas to help you carry out your grief work, but this is by no means an exhaustive list (see Appendix for further resources):

- See a grief counsellor or therapist – you might want to ask if they have experience with childlessness-related grief as many of us have found that therapists are not immune to the same uncon-scious prejudices as the rest of society. It's important too that you feel you 'click' with them when you first meet them; if you don't, keep looking. The quality of the relationship has a big impact on your experience, as this is an *intimate relationship* you're entering, albeit a professional one.

- Become a world-champion napper. Grief is exhausting physically, mentally and emotionally. If you imagine that your brain is being rewired with a whole new identity to take you forwards in life, perhaps you can stop feeling guilty about it and get napping. Try it without an alarm clock for the deluxe version.

- Spend time in nature. Nature is all about cycles of change, loss and rebirth. Spend a year really trying to notice the nature around you as it changes through the seasons. See how something always follows on from the end of something ... Be reassured that you are a part of nature and part of the same process. There will be new growth in your heart and in your life. You might even like to go on some sort of wilderness retreat, which can be a very cathar-tic process of getting in touch with your own 'wildness'.

- Engage in some form of creative practice to produce work inspired by your loss and in a nurturing, collective way where you can share that with others. It might be creative writing, music, sing-ing, sculpture, painting, etc. If such a group doesn't exist in your area, you might like to think about approaching a grief counsellor and asking them to start one, or starting your own with a group of other childless women. You can use the Gateway Women Meetup Groups for this, or start your own.

- Declutter your living space in the company of another childless woman with whom you can share the stories attached to the things you are releasing. You can then do the same for her. A wonderful guide to decluttering is Marie Kondo's *The Life-Changing Magic of Tidying*.[80]

- Meditation and mindfulness practices can be a good way to learn to pay attention to where our mind is running off to, and the stories that we are telling ourselves, some of which may be making us miserable. Learning to separate our consciousness from the grief-filled narrative running in our mind can be really helpful; it's also good for the opposite: leaning right into it and seeing what's really going on, and what lies beyond or behind it ...

- Yoga can be wonderful, although you may find doing it at home with a great video is preferable to attending classes, which can be a magnet for pregnant women. To avoid them I started going to Ashtanga yoga classes, as it's a pretty intensive form of yoga and not recommended for pregnant women. But then I moved areas and my new class had a female yoga teacher and of course *she* got pregnant!

- Watching films that make you laugh and cry can be powerful grief work. Some of us find that we don't have the ability to concentrate for a whole film at home during grief and I've found that going to the cinema works better for me. It's also quite liberating to let our emotions rip in a collaborative atmosphere. Tracey Cleantis has a 'Movie Rx' section at the end of each chapter of her book, *The Next Happy*,[81] if you'd like some inspiration.

- Mournful music that allows our sadness to rise to the surface and find expression can be helpful, particularly for those for whom tears don't seem to be coming easily at the moment. One of the women I've worked with recommended Pergolesi's 'Stabat Mater Dolorosa'. I find film scores, which track the emotional journey of the storyline, often move me to tears quite easily.

- Take up drumming and dance: traditional societies have used drumming, singing and dance as part of their grief journey and it's a wonderful way to move some of the physical aspects of grief through the body. Gabrielle Roth created a form of dance practice called 'Five Rhythms' (you absolutely don't need to be able to dance to do it!) and classes take place all over the world. It's a set sequence of five different 'tempos' and is a great way to release blocked energy. Grief doesn't just live in our thoughts …

- Attend a workshop or group for childless women. Gateway Women organises them, there are others listed in the Appendix and there are new organisations gradually forming all over the world. Keep an eye on the 'Resources' section of the Gateway Women website as I add to it whenever I hear of something that might help.

- Many women find keeping a journal helpful, although I found that because it wasn't a 'dialogue' (as no one but me was reading it) it didn't work for me. It wasn't until I started blogging that things began to shift, as women from all over the world were reading my thoughts and sharing their own. You can blog anonymously, which can be tremendously liberating, as so much of our thoughts and feelings around our childlessness seem to be socially unacceptable.

- Collect quotes on grief and grief recovery. I used to write down inspirational quotes on index cards, and choose one each day to prop up next to my bathroom mirror. Now I have a Pinterest board for this, which also means I can share them with others.[82] Alternatively, you can keep a special notebook or 'art journal' for them.

- Find out more about the lives of childless and childfree women around the world, both contemporary and historical. I have been building a gallery with mini-biographies of such women for a few years and now have more than 500. It's good to know that others have gone before us into this territory and have found a way through.

- Become part of an online community for childless women, such as the Gateway Women online community or others that are springing up now (see Appendix). Research has shown that 'silent' members who read but don't post get as much healing from it as those who post comments and take a more 'active' part.[83]

- Attend, listen to or watch comedy, whatever makes you really laugh. It's a great relief during grief. Developing a rather 'dark' sense of humour is also very common during grief and is a normal and healthy human response to distress. The darker the shadow, the brighter the light. (One word of warning on stand-up comedy shows: it now seems quite fashionable for male comics to talk about the highs and lows of parenthood, so check before you go!) There are some great comedy podcasts, and most comedians have something on their websites you can download.

- Taking care of a pet can be a wonderful outlet for our nurturing – both giving and receiving. For many childless women, nursing a pet from a rescue centre back to health and happiness has been a major part of their recovery. Others have found great reassurance in the way that our pets love us unconditionally when we feel at our most unlovable and like a burden to those around us. Research into Animal Assisted Therapy (AAT) has shown that the human–animal bond can be highly effective in supporting humans through the grief process, whether in the palliative care environ-ment or in the home.[84]

- Set up a Gateway Women reading group or Meetup in your area. It can be a social get-together in a coffee shop (or cocktail bar!), a picnic, dog-walking together, cultural outing or something more therapeutically minded where you meet up once a month (or weekly) to work through this book together. The relief of being amongst kindred spirits cannot be underestimated. One of the wonderful and surprising aspects of a Gateway Women Meetup is that because you know you're not going to be ambushed by any child-related talk, you don't necessarily *need* to talk about your childlessness, but instead can have a gloriously interesting and fun conversation about just about anything! A group of adult women *not* talking about children or childrearing can be a dynamic place to be.

- Take part in an online grief community such as Melody Beattie's 'Grief Club',[85] write your own blog about your grief, or comment on other grief-related blogs in order to get a dialogue going. This can be anonymous – whatever makes it possible for you to share your experience with others who understand and respond.

- Buddy up with another childless woman and work through this book together; you can connect through online communities at first and then progress to meeting up face to face.

- Read books about other women's recovery from childlessness and discuss them with other childless women, either online or in person.

- Become familiar with Kübler-Ross's Five Stages of Grief as they show up in all areas of life. Learning to name what you are experiencing with increasing precision will really help you process your grief.

- Supporting other childless women in *their* grief work can be profoundly healing. Perhaps offer your support to a woman who is creating a ritual, or a Meetup? Even the fairly minimal effort involved in sharing some of your experience with someone who is struggling in an online forum is enough to feel that we can be 'of use' and that can be very reassuring when we're grieving and may be feeling a bit 'useless'.

- Talk, talk, talk about your situation with other childless women who 'get it' until you're bored with talking about it. Boredom with talking about our story is a good sign that we've processed that part of our grief. Usually, our story 'shifts' at this point and we start to look at it in a different way. This is what's called 'processing' our grief. It's an ongoing process, though – each layer needs to be worked through.

- Listen, listen, listen to other childless women and be that non-judgemental, advice-free and empathetic sounding board that we all need to do our grief work.

Grieving is as individual as loving, so there may be ways that work for you that I haven't listed. If it allows you to communicate your experience and feel heard and understood in a non-judgemental and empathetic way; if perhaps it makes you cry healing tears that leave you feeling better not worse, then it's grief work.

EXERCISE 4
Doing Your Grief Work

Look back over each of Kübler-Ross's Five Stages of Grief in this chapter and note down how you have experienced, or are experiencing, each stage. Keep this with you over the next week and see if you can add to it as you become more aware of the different stages of grief and how they are showing up for you. Be gentle with yourself and don't worry if you're not sure where you are in the grief process. Just becoming aware that you are grieving may be all you need for things to start shifting.

This is not a test. It's about becoming a gentle witness to your own grief, so that you can work out what you need to do, and what support you'd like to get right now to continue your grief work.

Read through the 'What is Grief Work?' section and pick something to explore as part of your own grief recovery.

Reflections on Chapter 4

In this chapter, we've started exploring how grief over our childlessness has affected us and how it continues to do so. Depending on how much grief work you've done, this may all be new to you, or you may be relieved to discover that you're further along in the process than you realised.

However, living as we do in a culture that is in denial about grief and loss, and which often fails to recognise *our* loss at all, we may find that not only do we have more grief work to do, but that by allowing ourselves to grieve our childlessness, other ungrieved losses start surfacing too. It might be the dog that died when you were six or how you felt when your parents divorced. Each of us has a history of loss and if it's come up for healing, try not to push it down again. If the losses that begin to surface are deep ones from childhood, like the death of a parent or another major trauma, you may want to think about seeking the help of a bereavement or trauma therapist. Try not to panic about this because if the grief is coming up now then it is ready to heal you and you are ready to allow it. However, like all grief work, you cannot do it alone. This is not about you being too weak to deal with it, it's just that that's not how grief works – it needs understanding company. You may find that seeking the support of other childless women is enough, or you may wish to supplement that with other support. Trust yourself and the grief process. Grief is kind and gentle, but we can be rough and mean to ourselves. Grief wants to heal you, not hurt you. If you'd welcome the support of a trained counsellor or therapist for this, there are some resources I've gathered in the Appendix that might help you find someone who's right for you.

Learning the many different ways that grief can be experienced, and the many different ways we can support ourselves (and others) during this process, can feel a little overwhelming, like you're revising for some huge grief exam! However, please don't feel you need to become some kind of expert to do your grieving 'right'. The only thing necessary for your grieving is you, as your grief, like you, is totally unique. Nobody ever had to teach you how to fall in love – it was there inside you until the conditions came along to awaken it; it's the same with grief. Humans know how to grieve instinctively. Sometimes, the trick is as much getting out of our own way as anything else. Trust yourself, trust your grief. It'll get you to the other side of this dark period in your life.

If you did the 'Doing Your Grief Work' exercise, how did you find it? Often, women in my groups and workshops find learning about Kübler-Ross's Five Stages of Grief model a great help and having a way to name their feelings hugely relieving. 'I just thought I was going crazy,' is a not-uncommon response. Many of them (myself included) didn't know that what they were experiencing *was* grief. It's a good idea to reread this chapter whenever you get stuck and take action using some of the suggestions in 'What is Grief Work?' to obtain some relief and be able to move forward again. Learning to proactively work with grief rather than waiting for it to pass is a habit that will reap dividends for the rest of your life.

Bizarre as it may sound, have fun with your grief work! Laughter is a big part of recovery and the dark humour that grief can generate can be very healing, even if it does feel a bit 'shocking' at times!

If
childless women
are
CAREER WOMEN,
where are the
CAREER MEN
then?

CHAPTER 5

Liberating Yourself from the Opinions of Others

So, Have You Got Kids Then?

Once upon a time, if we went to the hairdresser, we'd be asked an innocuous social question such as, 'Been anywhere nice on holiday?' But these days, whether at the hairdresser, the bikini-waxing parlour, the dentist, a business conference or a party, the question often seems to be, 'So, have you got kids then?' or perhaps, 'So, how old are yours then?'

No doubt you've got your own horror story about being quizzed in public, but I think the most hurtful one I ever experienced was at my father-in-law's funeral with my soon-to-be ex-husband, out of rehab for the occasion. An elderly woman collared me to tell me 'how selfish' my generation were, 'too obsessed with their careers to have children'. The truth was that at this point, my husband and I had been trying to conceive for about nine years, and I'd never even met or spoken to this woman before. I still have no idea who she was. It was already a very upsetting day and she managed to make it a great deal worse.

It can also be really tough when people presume that I *do* have children, but that they're just not here at the moment. 'Isn't it great when they go back to school?' a woman might say to me at the beginning of the new school term at a supermarket checkout. Or, when it's presumed that we *chose* not to have them: 'Such a good idea not having kids – more trouble than they're worth!'

Finding the Right Answer

In my workshops, I sometimes do an exercise where women write down on one index card what they say when someone asks them if they have children, and on the other card what they *wished* they had the nerve to say if they're asked the common follow-up question, 'Why not?'

Here is a selection:

Do you have kids? (Some real and 'fantasy' answers)
No.
Nope. No kids, no pets, no houseplants . . .
No, do you?
No, only cats.
No, I forgot.
No, I'm like a vegetarian, but for kids.
No, but I've got a lizard.
No, I can barely look after myself . . .
No, but I am about to buy one.
No, some people don't and I'm not a weirdo.
Unfortunately not.
I don't think so . . .

Why not? (Some real and 'fantasy' answers)
Interesting question . . . Why do you ask?
Why did you choose to have children?
Because we couldn't.
I can't have them; I had an early menopause.
I had recurrent miscarriages.
The stork lost my address.
I didn't see motherhood as the be-all and end-all of my life's purpose.
Because sometimes life isn't fair.

Just like a lot of women, it didn't work out for me.

I never did find the right sperm donor, are you volunteering?

I met my husband late in life.

The number of women who wish they could say something along the lines of 'get lost' is really high, and the language can get pretty colourful! I haven't shared those here, but I'm sure you know what I mean ... What the intensity of this might show is how angry many of us feel about being put on the spot by this question which is, to most people, a 'safe' social opener. But not for us.

We also know that the likelihood of the person not feeling at ease with our 'difference' is quite high and that if they're asking this question, it nearly always means that they *do* have children ... and so therefore the chance is that we're *never* going to be part of 'their club'. In my experience it does seem to be very rare that a childless or childfree woman asks this question of others; most of us are too aware of how intrusive it can be.

However, if we put ourselves for a moment in the shoes of our unsuspecting inquisitors, they can't win, no matter <u>*what*</u> *they say about children.*

If they know it's a delicate area for us and avoid the topic of children like the plague, we might feel left out. And if they do talk about their children, on some days we might go ashen-faced and leave the room, but at other times we're happy to look at their holiday photos and laugh along with the cute antics of their kids. We might rail at them for their thoughtlessness or harangue them for not inviting us to their kids' parties. But more often than not, there'll just be an awkward silence and they'll find someone 'easier' to talk to. These are the social tumbleweed moments of childlessness, and learning to cope with them can make a huge difference to our daily life.

Although as many as one in five women in the UK and other developed countries don't have children, we need to remember that four out of five women do. We're the ones in the minority and we're the ones who have a problem with this question, so it's up to us to find a way to deal with it as best we can.

It's hard and it's unfair, I know – and when we're still grieving or having a 'griefy' moment, it's even harder. A good tactic is to have a few different answers that you feel comfortable using in different social situations, so you're as prepared as you can be. Perhaps you might find some inspiration from some of the answers above and try a few out? I find that these days I'm able to say, 'No, I couldn't have them,' without any great drama, and when I'm then asked, 'Why don't/didn't you adopt?' (often the next question!) I say, 'It wasn't an option for me,' again, without rancour. And unless it seems like an interesting opportunity to talk about the realities of modern childlessness, I gently steer the subject in a new direction – often by asking them a question about themselves. And on we go.

I have very few crash-and-burn social interactions around my childlessness any more, and I think this has a great deal to do with how at peace with it I feel myself. I've noticed that if someone seems to be trying to bait me using provocative comments about my 'selfishness' in not having children, for example, I leave the hook hanging these days. I'd rather save my energy for a conversation where I might be able to make a difference rather than, to paraphrase Shannon Alder, waste my time trying to explain myself to someone committed to misunderstanding me.[86] It's also the reason why I don't read the comments online posted underneath articles I've written, although they can be good to show people who think that I'm 'making it up' that some people can be cruel and prejudiced towards childless women.

I feel differently about my childlessness on different days. Sometimes, after a busy day out and about, I'm thrilled to arrive home to a quiet house with just the cat to feed, and at other times I simply can't quite believe that this is how my life turned out.

Perhaps some of the hardest moments are coming home having been embedded in someone else's family life for a few days – I've named that coming-back-into-my-own-life feeling an 'intimacy hang-over' (inspired by Brené Brown's 'vulnerability hangover'[87]) and since I've found a way to name it, it helps it to pass more quickly.

On my now very rare griefy days, I've learned not to try and 'pull my socks up' emotionally but to show myself some self-compassion, drop the 'story' I might be building up around the often very physical sensa-tion of grief and allow it to pass through me, like a storm. Respecting my grief by giving it space and time has proven to be the very best way to move through it quickly. These days, the weather can shift again in a couple of hours ... or at most a couple of days. I really don't mind my griefy days anymore; after all, I used to have griefy years!

All of us childless women are accidental pioneers.
We didn't choose this difference, this role. Consequently,
we haven't been preparing for it throughout our lives
and so may need to actively seek out and practise
the skills needed to cope with it.

I do understand that it's also hard on men who wanted to be fathers, but it seems that they are not exposed to judgemental remarks with the same relentless frequency as women, although that also depends on which country you're in – from interviewees for this book I've learned that pronatalism varies hugely from country to country. From Canada, John wrote:

I'm asked most often at work – if there is someone new at work
they always ask, so I probably get asked about once a month.
I think I get asked pretty equally by both men and women; they
both have the same kind of question: 'Do you have kids?' I usually
just say, 'No, it's a long story,' or, 'We tried and it didn't work out,'

*that sort of thing. Most people stop talking about it pretty quickly
after that but some people want to know more details. I'll say
then that we tried a lot of different ways (natural conception, IVF,
adoption) and then usually even the talkier ones stop asking.*

John: 42, Married, Canada

Although an older man without children may be viewed with a
certain suspicion as some kind of potential child molester, which is
not something women have to cope with, often it is presumed that they
just don't have children *yet*. Male factor infertility, being childless by
relationship or any of the many other reasons that might be involved in
a man's childlessness are rarely considered. Nor does it seem to occur
to most that involuntary childlessness might be a source of great pain
and grief for men too.

The Taboo of Childlessness

There seems to be no 'acceptable' way to talk about childlessness,
either voluntary or involuntary. It's a taboo and, like all taboos, the
way it's policed is that talking about it is seen as shameful and embarrassing. No one wants to risk raising the subject with us in case they
embarrass us (a mild form of shame) or we embarrass them. Childless
women often stay silent on the subject too, even with other women
who don't have children, 'just in case'.

---

*Nobody talks about childlessness, so it's never a
topic of conversation. And the longer this emotional
policing continues, the more shame attaches itself to
the subject and it becomes even harder to talk about.
That's how taboos work.*

It only takes two people to start breaking a social taboo: one to talk
about it and another to listen and be changed by that conversation. For

some reason, I am one of the women in our generation who has chosen to break this taboo, and I'm liberating others to do the same. It's a bit like *The Emperor's New Clothes* – the story in which the child points out the truth (that the emperor is naked) and this allows everyone else to admit what they knew all along but didn't dare say.

> *In my experience, people prefer to keep conversations light and superficial. If they think for a moment about how they might feel if they couldn't have children, they realise it's a potentially emotional topic. So they steer clear!*
>
> Jenni: 40, Single, Australia

Homosexuality was described at Oscar Wilde's trial as 'The love that dare not speak its name'[88] and, in some ways, I think 'coming out' as childless or childfree can feel a bit similar. In fact, a lesbian childless woman I know told me that for her, coming out as childless was actually harder. I'm pretty sure that our friends, family and society as a whole might be shocked to know that this is how we feel, and might even try to deny it vociferously, but until they've walked a day in our shoes, it's really hard to 'see' the taboo of childlessness; it's culturally invisible, although hopefully not for much longer. It has only taken a generation to see some positive change in attitudes towards the LGBT community and I hope that we can do the same for childlessness. We just need to stick together, speak out, and be prepared for some people to find our honesty challenging, at first.

> *Opening up about childlessness, when it wasn't a choice and you've bought into the idea that this makes you 'less than', means to make yourself very vulnerable and you might get hurt in the process. Therefore, many decide not to talk about it and cover it under a thick blanket of strict silence. So, in my view, a topic only becomes a problem, a 'social taboo', if I myself refuse to talk about it because I am scared of the reactions that might follow.*
>
> Ada: 38, Living with Partner, Germany/USA

One of my dearest friends (who is a mother) came to a public talk I gave to a group of Gateway Women on International Women's Day in March 2012. She was there to support me personally as it was the largest public talk I'd given at that point, but what struck her most was the way the women in the audience behaved. A childless documentary filmmaker wanted to film my talk, but none of the women in the audience were prepared to be seen on camera (even the backs of their heads). They were too scared that someone they knew might see the film and know that they were struggling with their childlessness (or potential childlessness). My friend, as a mother, had never heard women share their stories like this: their shame, isolation, depression, suicidal fantasies, stigma, grief and anger; she had no idea. The fact that these articulate, capable, intelligent women refused to allow themselves to be filmed, as if they had committed a crime, completely shocked her. She had no idea how shaming it felt to be a childless woman and although she'd heard me talk about it she didn't really *believe* it until she saw it with her own eyes.

'As a Mother ...'

Being a mother (whatever 'kind' of mother you are) gives a woman instant status; it's perhaps part of the reason why socially disadvantaged teenage girls become mothers. How many times have you seen a woman interviewed or mentioned in the news as, 'Mother of four, woman X, says ...'? By being a mother, these women are automatically given the status of grown-up women with an opinion that matters. I'm not saying that their opinion *doesn't* matter, but that the voice of mothers carries a disproportionate weight compared to that of non-mothers in our culture right now.

We're constantly bombarded with photos and news items about celebrity mothers and parents in the news, for whatever reason, being described as 'mother of two', 'grandmother of six', 'father to

two little boys'! What's the other side to that, a news item that
states, 'Childless woman blown up, but who cares anyway?'!
Marianne: 63, Married, UK

After all, how would *we* understand anything? 'You're not a mother, you wouldn't understand,' is the hurtful unspoken, and sometimes spoken, belief. And indeed, perhaps in *some* cases we might not. But not *all*.

We're all human. All experience is valid.
And <u>no one</u> has a monopoly on understanding.

The gift of empathy (literally 'feeling into') is what makes it possible for non-blood-related humans to live together in society. It makes civilisation possible. We all, to a greater or lesser degree, have the capacity to imaginatively feel what others' lives are like. We don't have to actually *live* those lives to perceive what it might be like for them. After all, this is how art and literature work: we imagine ourselves in another's shoes. It is one of the gifts of humanity and it is not one that childless women are incapable of. Considering that so many of us spent years dreaming of becoming mothers, we've had plenty of time to imagine how motherhood would be.

I'm very aware of, for example, politicians constantly talking about
'hard-working families', which drives me bonkers as I am literally
screaming at the television or radio, saying, 'What about me and
all the contributions that I make too?!'
Laura: 47, Single, UK

The power of a mother's love for her child has a fierceness that I will never experience first-hand. But I have a mother, I was a child once and I've been passionately in love. If I connect the unconditional love I have for my mother with the passionate intensity of romantic love, I think I can *imagine* what parental love might feel like. And therefore I can *imagine* how a love of that intensity and permanence might motivate a mother to behave in certain ways.

But how much time, if any, do mothers and others spend wondering what it's like to be us – to be a childless woman in a motherhood-obsessed culture?

What we ask for is that the gift of imaginative empathy be sent *our* way too. Our experience as childless women is valid and not something to be pushed out of mind as 'distasteful'. For one reason or another, around 20 per cent of all women will not become mothers, possibly many more in generations to come; it's no longer acceptable for us to be treated as freaks of nature.

How Our Own Family Responds to Our Childlessness

The way that childless women can be treated by their family of origin is often an area of great pain and confusion for the women I've worked with. There is sometimes a sense of deep betrayal that those who are meant to be there for us aren't, and that some of the most cutting comments and harshest exclusions can occur within the family setting. Perhaps some of the hottest areas are relationships between mothers and childless daughters, relationships between siblings (particularly sisters) when one has children and one doesn't, and issues around how parents treat those siblings.

> *The silence around my childlessness has been very strong in my family of origin. Nobody has ever asked me about it or showed any empathy and I experienced very insensitive treatment in earlier years. Nowadays I bring it up and include it in conversations, particularly with the younger members of the family, who seem more willing to talk about it, perhaps because it is affecting more of their generation.*
>
> Tilda: 64, Married, New Zealand

I came to a deeper understanding of why some mothers (perhaps including our own) might find it difficult to empathise with us as a result of a conversation with a dear girlfriend of mine. She'd been reading my blog and could see that I was in deep distress over my childlessness. She explained that the only way she could empathise with me was to imagine how she'd feel if her own child had died, and that when she did so, the feeling was so overwhelming it was very hard to stay with it. It was an extraordinarily helpful thing for her to share with me, as it helped me to understand why so few mothers are able to fully empathise with us − it takes them to one of the darkest places they can imagine; a fear that they carry with them all the time and which they do their best *not* to think about ... And then, if we remember that the very person we are asking for this level of empathy from may be our *own* mother, and that she'd need perhaps to imagine the feeling of losing *us*, the very daughter speaking with her, perhaps we can begin to understand the kind of emotional gymnastics we are expecting from them.

> *My family, knowing I have always wanted children, have never asked*
> *me how I feel. We are just not close like that. They will sometimes*
> *make a joke of my life, which hurts. My mum seems to say something*
> *to me every time I see her that either rips my heart out, or rubs my*
> *face in it. She's not a malicious woman, just insensitive to me.*
>
> Jenni: 40, Single, Australia

However, empathy for our own mothers' difficulties aside, perhaps what is hard for us is that what we get in place of the empathy that we crave is often judgement, comparisons or crass 'advice'. Judgements such as, 'Well, you *would* go to university!' (even though they had encouraged us) or comparisons such as, 'Well, your sister didn't have any problem finding a husband!' (not allowing for luck in such matters), or advice such as, 'Why don't you have a baby on your own? I'll help you look after it,' (when perhaps the mothering you received is a contributing factor to your childlessness and you'd struggle to leave a pet with her ...).

Although what is said or unsaid can be very hard to deal with, some of the toughest stuff that can come up is in the way that childless daughters are treated within the family dynamic, and which appears to show that in some way they are considered 'less important', even 'less adult', than their siblings who are parents. For example, when going home for big holidays or family events, childless women often find themselves being turfed out of their room to sleep on the sofa or blow-up bed so that a couple or their children can have 'her' room. I've even heard of one woman in her fifties being put in a tent in the garden so that her young niece could have her bed! This is usually done without consultation and when the childless daughter is shocked and hurt, she's often told she's being 'selfish' or 'too sensitive' or that 'it's silly to only have one person in that room', without an awareness that her feelings have very little to do with the accommodation arrangements, but are rather about what it communicates to her about how her family value her ...

> *They all know I wanted a family of my own. They all sympathise in their own ways, but none of them really empathise and there is a key difference there. I refuse now to allow myself to be compromised by family, e.g. sleeping on the sofa or on the floor in a room, etc. But I do know that there is a difference in the way I am looked at, because I'm not married or with a family, although they wouldn't see it this way.*
>
> Claude: 44, Single, UK

Other hurtful snubs include big family decisions about wills, estates and legacies being made only in consultation with those that have children, and estates being divided equally between children and grandchildren. Another issue can be parents who feel able to travel to the other side of the world to visit their grandchildren, but who consistently refuse to drive an hour to see their childless daughter, instead expecting her to always do the travelling. The childless daughter therefore rarely gets to be the 'host' and have her home and her way of life witnessed and experienced by her family. Such things may seem petty, but they can build up into a pattern of 'not mattering' that can cause a deep hurt which, over time, can become a festering resentment and even lead to family estrangements. And because so much of this behaviour is unconscious on the part of the family, when they *are* called on it, they think it's quite natural and acceptable and that the childless woman is being 'unreasonable'. What's playing out here are the deep roots of the social status quo (derived from patriarchal values), which all of us, men *and* women, have been brought up with, and which assigns a mature woman's 'value' according to her status as a partner and/or mother. If you're over forty and neither of these things, treating you like a second-class citizen is what all of us have been conditioned to think of as 'natural'. Until, that is, it's you on the receiving end and you can see it's a form of apartheid – another way of 'othering' us.

For many women, simply finding out that it's not just *their* family who can behave this way can come as a huge relief. Although it may not be easy or possible to shift these dynamics, talking about them with other childless women and swapping tips on what works, and how to put boundaries down around certain aspects, can really help. However, something I absolutely *don't* recommend is attempting to have these kinds of negotiations with your family members during (or just before) big family gatherings (when everyone's already stressed) and also not to do so until you've had a chance to do some grief work. It's good to have had a chance to explore some of your heated feelings with other childless women *before* you tackle it at source because, if it ends in a fight and a crying jag, it may just be used to back up their point of view that you're being 'unreasonable' and 'oversensitive'! This is a battle you need to train for as it's not really about you, it's about our culture's deepest conditioning about 'what is a family' and 'what is a woman'.

When you're ready, one way to open this area up for conversation with your family is to share an article about coming to terms with childlessness from a newspaper that your family respect. This can often carry more weight at first than your own opinion, especially if you're already on the back foot in terms of status in your family. This can also make it easier to discuss, as you can then talk about 'the article' rather than yourself.

Being Childless at Work

As if dealing with our childlessness in our family wasn't challenging enough, it's often tough at work too. From the endless round of pregnancy announcements, baby shower collections and meet-my-baby workplace visits, to the joke that is most corporate organisations' 'female-friendly' policies (mostly 'mother-friendly') and coping with the extra workload (and not being expected either to mind or be paid for it) when mothers have to duck out of work early or go on maternity leave, being childless in the modern workplace is not easy for the childless or childfree adult – woman or man.

> *It is very usual among my colleagues to think that you don't have a life if you don't have a husband and/or children, so they think your time is also available for them. You can be the last to leave the office (as you do not have to pick up your children from school); you can be the last to choose the vacation period, etc. They take you for granted.*
>
> Salome: 50, Single, Spain

There are two big issues here: grief and fairness. The grief is personal and we each have to find our way through with the support of other childless women and by doing our grief work. The unfairness, however, is a workplace issue and it's one that we need to start speaking up about.

In June 2014 a new law came into force in the UK to make it possible for everyone to request 'flexible working arrangements'[89] from their employers, not just parents and carers. The year before, an interview I gave in a British newspaper speaking candidly about the issues childless women face in the workplace went round the world in a flash, and I was even live on Australian breakfast TV! Once again, it seemed that I was articulating what many of us may have experienced, but which it's still unacceptable to voice. I wrote that:

> It's impossible to argue that your life outside work is as important as the needs of a small child, and complaining about it seems 'unsisterly' [...] There's an unbelievable permissiveness towards mothers at work. If they're bombarding their colleagues with child-related talk all day, it's deemed acceptable, but if women without children talk about their lives in the same way, we're seen as self-absorbed.[90]

Interestingly, when the new law was due to come into force, I was invited onto *Today*, the UK's most prestigious morning radio news show, to discuss the issue.[91] Even though I framed my argument as one of 'fairness', it was interesting how the interviewer wanted to steer the discussion towards one of 'childless women versus mothers', which is absolutely not how I see it! I totally support women's rights to have children *and* have a job; I've got no problem with that at all. What I resent is that employers are using the taboo of childlessness to push the extra work created by some mothers' uneven presence in the workplace onto their childless colleagues without this being recognised or compensated for. We're mostly expected to quietly 'suck it up' and, if we complain, we're seen as being 'bitter' about our childlessness.

Some of the issues we face are structural, they're not always emotional, although when we raise the former, we'll usually be accused of the latter! But until we come together and form a united front about such things, individually it's very easy for us to lose heart and back down, or never pluck up the courage to say anything at all.

> *As for bringing babies into work as some sort of badge of honour –*
> *it makes me steaming mad! Although I think a lot about talking to*
> *HR, I am hesitant about drawing attention to myself.*
>
> Natasha: 53, Single, UK

And it seems it doesn't matter how high up the food chain you go either. In 2008, a stray microphone caught an American governor's remark about Governor Janet Napolitano as Barack Obama's choice for Secretary of Homeland Security as a good one because she 'has no family' and the job requires someone who 'has no life ... she can devote, literally, 19–20 hours a day to it'.[92]

Challenging the Stereotypes of Childless Women

While the respect and empathy we crave from others may still be some time coming, for the moment we can at least change the way we feel about *ourselves*. Just because the culture currently only has a limited set of restrictive and reductive stereotypes for us to fit into, we don't actually have to comply ...

This is how all change happens: from the inside out.

When I ask childless women in my groups and workshops to think of as many archetypes, names or roles as they can for older, childless women, here are the ones they most commonly come up with:

- Spinster, old maid
- Crazy old cat lady (often smelly too!)
- Career woman
- Dried-up old bag, bat or hag
- Maiden aunt
- Lesbian
- Wicked or evil stepmother
- Witch
- And so on ...

Depressing, isn't it! However, upon closer inspection, I've discovered that if we group these negatives into 'themes', something interesting starts to appear: suppressed power.

It would seem that each one of these negative archetypes, when turned on its head, reveals what this shaming is really all about – the suppression of feminine power.

But why should this power be so threatening that it has to be shamed into silence, into inaction? Perhaps it's because if the power that childless women potentially possess were to be used purposefully and respected culturally it would undermine one of the central planks of patriarchy – namely that men are 'in charge' because they're inherently more capable? When perhaps the reality might be that the reason men have historically been so is because they haven't been bringing up children ...

THE HIDDEN POWER WITHIN CHILDLESS WOMEN STEREOTYPES

Stereotypes	Power-types
Spinster, old maid	An unpartnered mature childless woman. *Independent, competent, confident, creative, resourceful, educated, financially independent, free, liberated and wordly-wise. Powerful.*
Crazy cat lady	An unpartnered mature childless woman who may (but not always) live alone and has a cat. *Independent, sensitive, empathic, practical, perceptive, nurturing, free, attuned, generous and self-sufficient. Powerful.*

Career woman	A mature childless woman who works for a living.
	Educated, financially independent, self-assured, resourceful, free, adventurous, savvy, competent, liberated, astute and courageous. Powerful.
Dried-up old bag, bat or hag	A mature post-menopausal childless woman.
	Wise, confident, capable, outspoken, liberated, self-aware, sexually knowledgeable, articulate and open. Powerful.
Maiden aunt	A childless older woman with warm and friendly relationships with children not her own.
	Independent, knowledgeable, generous, kind, resourceful and financially independent. Powerful.
Lesbian	A childless woman who prefers women as sexual and life partners.
	Self-determining, self-aware, liberated, rebellious, independent and astute. Powerful.
Wicked or evil stepmother	A childless stepmother.
	Understanding, wise, kind, nurturing, generous, supportive and practical. A powerful influence on children not her own.
Witch	An outspoken childless older woman.
	Confident, courageous, fierce, knowledgeable, self-aware and unapologetic. Powerful.

Reductive archetypes are not *exclusively* used for childless women; we all use them and they act as a useful form of social shorthand. From the 'yummy mummy' to the 'helicopter parent', mothers get labelled too, but rarely do their labels contain the spite and shaming power that childless women's archetypes do. Apart from being branded 'a bad mother' perhaps.

In fact, very few of those stereotypes used to diminish childless women are used to our face, except perhaps 'career woman'. However, whether used *to* us or *about* us, as a tool of ideological control such negative archetypes have done a good job of making older childless women feel so ashamed of themselves that they've felt uncomfortable embracing the power and freedom that their situation allows.

> *I frankly get angry when someone tries to shame me – what nerve! However, I understand the shame feelings. Shame is an instrument of control. I think we are shamed and treated as a disappointment and as defective as women because being childless we now are free women, and freedom for women is a taboo.*
>
> Margot: 67, Married, USA

By tuning into the 'light' side of these archetypes we can begin to claim this power in our own lives, and direct it as we see fit. It's ours to own and shape as suits our personality and life circumstances, not there for others to shame, silence and belittle us with. It may take time to believe this but if you consider how believing the alternative makes you feel, maybe it's not such a bad idea?

Spinsters

Whereas 'bachelor' is a term that implies a future, 'spinster' is one loaded with failure. It's as if all possibilities of happiness, of things turning out OK, are quashed by the word 'spinster'.

This is ironic because the original fourteenth-century term simply denoted a woman who was unmarried and had the profession of 'spinner' – some of the first 'career women' in fact. Spinsters were often additional breadwinners for their families, as they were able to work from home and combine it with taking care of other members of the family. It wasn't until the Industrial Revolution in Britain in the late eighteenth and early nineteenth centuries, and the way that it drastically changed family and community life, that the term developed its current pejorative meaning.[93]

These days, spinster carries the unstated prefix 'bitter'. It denotes a woman who is presumed to have been too stupid, unattractive or ambitious to hold onto a partner and/or have a baby during her fertile years and, moreover, for that to be the most defining feature about her, outweighing all others. Whereas just a generation ago, being an unmarried mother was to be the social outcast, now it's the single, childless woman over forty who carries the weight of shame. Yet, for some women this is not a situation they chose, but rather one that they've ended up in because they've made intelligent, honourable choices and behaved with decency and morality towards others. Some of them may have cared for vulnerable family members through their fertile years, have refrained from getting pregnant 'accidentally' without a partner's consent, have said no to marriage with partners that they didn't feel they could wholeheartedly commit to, have worked hard as members of their families, in workplaces and communities, and have contributed to society as taxpayers. The notion that such women are somehow 'failures' is obscene.

> Recognising that much of my grief was tied to fear about being on my own, unloved, etc., combined with negative social ascriptions about being a childless woman, did not come to awareness until much later for me. When this clicked, and when I began to question and reject those negative beliefs, my happiness returned. I'm busy reclaiming the term 'spinster' for myself now and I use it all the time.
>
> Eimear: 44, Single, Ireland

With more and more of us remaining single, not all of us by choice, the idea that a single childless woman is some kind of 'Bridget Jones' character is both unflattering and inaccurate. In the UK, 10 per cent of adults aged 25–44 now live alone, five times the rate recorded in 1973.[94] And in the US, it has risen from 17 per cent in 1970 to 27 per cent of households in 2012, with more than half of those being women (this data includes single parents and divorced/widowed women). It appears to be a global trend, with one-person households having risen by 30 per cent in the last 10 years.[95] It's really time to appreciate that single adults are a feature of modern life, and not some kind of aberration to be looked down upon from the safe perch of 'coupledom'. A piece of 2011 American research[96] showed it is singles (or 'solos', which I prefer as it has a much less judgemental tone to it) who, compared to their married peers, contribute the greatest amount of support to their parents (both men and women), are more connected to the lives of their siblings, nieces and nephews, are more involved in their local community through voluntary work and visiting neighbours and are also more active in local and national political life than those who are married.[97] So much for selfish, huh?

'Singlism' and 'matrimania' are two terms coined by the American academic researcher and writer Bella DePaulo, whose rigorous research analysis shows how the bias against singles persists 'in the workplace, the marketplace, the media, in religion, in pseudoscience, in laws and policies, and in our everyday lives'.[98] Once we begin to open our eyes to how our culture persists in portraying the 'spinster' as a sad, lonely woman, and instead start to realise that it's up to us if we buy into it, the door is open to enjoying the benefits that being solo brings as well as learning not to be hard on yourself for its challenges. There has never been a better time to be a solo and childless women. It's not *Bridget Jones* and it's not *Sex in the City*; it's life – complicated, sometimes wonderful, regularly challenging, perhaps at times lonely and often incredibly liberating.

Crazy Old Cat Lady

More than maybe any other stereotype, the 'crazy old cat lady' seems to have the power to strike the most fear into the hearts of childless women. So much so that those who take pleasure in their pets, as I do (and always have), may try to hide that from people in case they are ridiculed. In the Gateway Women online community, I started a section called 'Furbabies' and within hours the community timeline was a solid wall of fluff. Yet these same women would never have shared these pictures with their friends on Facebook because of the shame they'd feel. 'Oh, so these are baby substitutes?!' some people will sneer unkindly. What's going on here?

My feeling is that it may have something to do with the fact that nurturing our pets is extremely rewarding, and that the love and affection that our pets give us in return is not something we 'deserve'. After all, we're meant to be miserable outcasts, not happy pet owners. The way that our pets bond with us in just the same way as they do with other humans perhaps also unconsciously points out that childless women are actually no different from other people. It may be that some mothers, feeling perhaps a bit stitched up by pronatalism and finding parenting, for all the social approval they get, much less rewarding and meaningful that they expected, may unconsciously resent us having this pleasure?

I used to be really sensitive to the whole 'furbaby' thing ... until I realised that was just my own shame speaking. For example, for a long time I wanted to get a bike-trailer for my dog (I'm a keen cyclist and this opened up possibilities for me), but I worried about what people would think about me. This is odd because I don't normally worry about what people think of me ... childlessness goes deep, though. Once I began to emerge from my grief and, thanks to the Gateway Women online community, started to understand the societal influence on my feelings, I dropped the shame and now embrace being the 'crazy dog lady'. I love people peering into my trailer to find a border collie and not a baby. In fairness, the reaction has only ever been positive, but I no longer care about any judgements that may or may not be made in private.

Sam: 41, Married, UK

I remember a conversation I overheard at a drinks party during the last couple of years of my 'still hopeful' period. A beautiful and talented single childfree-by-choice woman was being pursued by a man who didn't seem to be getting anywhere. In frustration he blurted out, 'If you're not careful, you're going to end up as one of those old women living on her own with loads of cats!' And her answer, to my delight and amazement was, 'If everything goes to plan.' I laughed out loud and it lodged in my brain as something so unusual I couldn't forget it. It's taken me years to understand how radical it was of her, and how much I admire her for it.

The fact is, there's absolutely nothing to fear about living on your own or having pets. It's not everyone's choice but neither is it such a terrible fate. After all, if you're content on your own and have animals around you to nurture your spirit, what's the big deal? It's power, of course. Because a woman like this is one who has unplugged from the patriarchy – she doesn't need to be someone's wife or mother to be happy, and, as I said earlier, that's a threat to the status quo. So the very thought of it has been made into a shaming stereotype. Now, I'm not saying that every old woman who lives on her own with cats is happy about that. But neither is every old woman living in her adult children's spare bedroom and having her freedom curtailed by unwanted child-care duties for her grandchildren, whilst enduring blaring music and slamming doors. Both are stereotypes that whitewash the individual reality of each woman's situation.

The crazy cat lady stereotype is something that I both fear and look forward to. I can't have pets in my life at the moment but one day I really hope to, and I have a real affinity for cats, so I believe being a cat lady is my destiny. However, the thought of other people's judgement makes me feel sad and kind of weary – it is the prospect of all of those conversations in my future, and all of those unspoken judgements about me. But then I find myself feeling a kind of defiant satisfaction in embracing the stereotype and saying 'f**k it' to them all.

Amelie: 41, Single, UK

Wrapped up in the fear of becoming the crazy old cat lady are other fears – of losing our mind when we're old, of being alone and having no one to care for us and all the worries of old age that lurk at the edges of adult consciousness. Perhaps one of the reasons that this stereotype has such a strong hold is because right now just about everyone's scared of getting old and what's going to happen. The old way of being old doesn't work anymore and a new way of doing it hasn't yet taken hold. Perhaps by projecting their own fear of ageing back onto us with the help of this stereotype, parents may feel protected from it for a moment?

If we look the crazy cat lady stereotype full in the face and own both its light and shadowy aspects, perhaps we can see that all things considered, it might not actually be such a bad a way to live out our twilight years? After all, having learned to live with childlessness, we're probably more equipped to deal with the isolation and issues of old age than many parents. They may have children, but we'll have developed internal resources and a strong social network to support ourselves by then.

Career Woman

'Career woman' is a term applied to older childless women who work for a living. It's a term that implies that the woman has *chosen* her career over having a family and thus has proved herself to be 'not all that maternal', which is code for not a 'real' woman. Although you do have to wonder what other kind of woman there could possibly be apart from real ones!

> *I have been called a 'career girl', which I have to say always makes me laugh as I have only had 'jobs', as my 'career plan' from a very young age had always been to get married and have a family. So I find it particularly irritating when people say that to me as it's so untrue!*
>
> Laura: 47, Single, UK

Now, there are indeed women who recognise that if they want to get to the top of their profession, they're possibly going to have to forgo having children. And if they make that choice, however tinged with regret, it *is* a legitimate choice. Dame Janet Baker, the world-famous British opera singer, said in a 2012 interview in the *Guardian*, 'I knew, energy wise, that I couldn't both bring up children and have a career. And that has never been a decision I have regretted.'[99] However, not all of us have the interest, talent or support to get to the top of our profession, and even childless women doing what they would describe as 'jobs' are called career women. And of course, one does have to wonder how many top male opera singers have had to make the same choice . . .

> *Because most people succeed in having children, those who don't are seen as 'different' and don't fit the social mould. It's never explicit, but what winds me up more than anything is the assumption that I'm a career woman instead. I AM NOT defined by my work.*
>
> Claude: 44, Single, UK

An Irish radio station once interviewed me, hot on the heels of a newspaper article about Gateway Women.[100] The male presenter referred to me on air as a 'career woman' and I corrected him. 'No,' I said, 'I'm a woman who works. I wanted a family and it didn't work out for me. And in the years that it didn't work out, I carried on working as I needed to earn a living. I did not *choose* work over a family. And now that I've been consistently working, without much interruption, for the last thirty years, it looks like a career.' I could practically hear him rustling his researcher's notes, wondering how a sob story about a woman without children had gone all 'feminist' on him!

For those of us who are what is now being called 'socially infertile', to be called a 'career woman' is to imply a degree of choice about the situation that often wasn't there.

The fact is, in order to succeed in the workplace, many more women have become highly educated and often don't even start their professional life until their early to mid-twenties. By the time they've learned the skills of their profession and have moved up the ladder, they're thirty. At this point, they're still confident of their attractiveness in the marriage market and hope to get married and have children in the next couple of years. But now they face a situation that, as yet, is not really being talked about – 'marrying up'.

We are living through a transitional time in the relationship between the sexes and carrying some old paradigms and conventions into entirely new situations, where they make an uneasy fit; marrying up is one of them. In the days when marriage was a woman's only chance to improve her economic status, choosing a partner of a higher social or economic status was a key ambition. Think of Jane Austen novels if you want to recall how crucial it used to be. And the more beautiful or accomplished the young woman, the 'better' she could do for herself.

However, as women went into higher education and the professions in vastly greater numbers, this was *not* matched by a corresponding increase in men doing the same. So now we have a generational situation where many *more* women are looking to choose partners from the same limited pool of high-status men. It is not that there is a drought of 'good men', as some women believe, but that there is a flood of 'good women', so much so that in New York City, there are currently '100,000 more women than men who are college educated and under thirty-five, a fact not usually reported when dating-related issues are discussed in the media'.[101]

Add to this that a 'high-status' man will often prefer to partner with a young, attractive woman with plenty of time left on her fertility clock, and we have a situation where many women around the age of forty are finding themselves still unpartnered, or with men who are not 'right' to have a family with.

This effect does not work entirely in men's favour, though; it only works for high-status men. 'Lower-status' men (once called blue-collar workers), who traditionally would have had no difficulty finding a wife, are similarly being left unpartnered. As many of the women from their own background have become executives and doctors rather than the secretaries and nurses they may have been a generation ago, they are often no longer interested in dating or marrying them.

However, as professional single women move into their mid to late thirties, held fast in the grip of babymania, some of them reluctant-ly begin to consider these lower-status men as someone they could 'settle for'. The men, perhaps bitter and sore after years of rebuffs and loneliness, are quite likely to reject the women as being 'over the hill' just to get even. And anyway, who can blame them for not wanting to start a family with someone who's possibly always going to resent them for being 'not quite good enough'? Think of Miranda in the TV series *Sex and the City*, who has a baby with Steve, a 'good man'. But so many of their problems as a couple are due to their differing status – as professional versus blue-collar, college-educated versus street-smart.

There are so many interlocking factors that lead to childlessness – unconscious behaviours and outdated beliefs, mixed with our new way of living and working. We all need to remember that it's only fifty years since we started this experiment after many thousands of years of women being reliant on men economically, and pregnancy being mostly out of women's control.

In the meantime, we need to start talking about how these changes are affecting everyone, both men *and* women. We need not take all the blame on our shoulders, nor presume that all men are happy with the unintended consequences of their choices either. Childless women are an easy target because we already bear the shame of the childless taboo, but we don't need to take *all* the blame for the fallout from perhaps the biggest shift in relationships between men and women since we moved from the earlier matrilineal to our current patriarchal social structure ten thousand years ago.[102]

Aunts and Godmothers

Whilst many of us have nephews, nieces and godchildren, not all of us are as actively involved in their lives as the stereotype of the doting aunt or godmother would seem to suggest. It implies, once again, that we 'lack' something and that we will only fulfil it through a vicarious involvement with other people's children. This in turn reinforces the idea that only children can bring meaning into our lives, which isn't true, although it's such a prevalent one that it's hard to believe it's just an idea, not a truth. It's also not the case that all of us get asked to be godmothers. Although I have been asked five times, and have been greatly flattered on each occasion, some childless women have never been asked at all.

> *I feel sad about not being asked to be a godmother ... It feels like no one thinks I am fit for it, even though I believe I'd be a great role model for their children. I feel a bit jealous too about friends who already have children and who are being asked.*
>
> Celeste: 39, Single, French Canada

There's absolutely nothing wrong with being involved in the lives of the children around us – Melanie Notkin, founder of Savvy Auntie, has coined a great word for it: 'childful'[103] – but it's the act of being *defined* by that involvement that I take issue with.

Being an active aunt or godmother is not a way of compensating for our childlessness; it is an act of love and care for others. To suggest that our love for the young people in our life is some kind of compensation mechanism is an insult to all of those women involved in the lives of children not their own. Ours is a loving and voluntary choice, not purely a way to fulfil a biological need. And it is one that, no matter how important it is to the children, can be revoked by the parents at any time, which can add a real sense of powerlessness that can echo the grief of involuntary childlessness. It is not always an easy relationship, although that's often how it's portrayed.

> *I worry in particular about how dependent my role as an aunt is on other people's permission; my brother has two children who I love dearly, but his relationship with his wife is fractious, at best. If he ever leaves (and he talks about leaving regularly), I really fear for my relationship with my niece and nephew. As an aunt, you have no legal right to access.*
>
> Anna: 32, Married, UK

Wrapped up in the doting aunt stereotype of the fussy older child-less woman clucking around children, liberally dispensing treats and patting them on the head, is a kind of neutralising, desexing patron-isation. The stereotypical childless aunt is not portrayed as some kind of *va-va-voom* exciting, glamorous grown-up, but rather as a sexless, shapeless, harmless (free) babysitter. This stereotype devalues both the real contribution so many childless women (blood-related or not) make to the lives of children and the nature of the relationship. We are not default babysitters and cake-makers; we are that 'village' that children need as they grow to maturity. We offer a different take on life from their mothers and peers, one that they seek and value us for.

> *I'm aunt and godmother to all five of my sister's children and also godmother to two of my friend's children. I am a fun auntie and I'm also trusted with their care, and luckily my sister has always taken the view that it's important that they have someone to turn to other than their parents, should they need to. My sister often confides in me if she thinks the children are worried about something but won't tell her what, and I might then spend a bit of time with them and sometimes they do open up. My experience as godparent to my friends' children, however, is different. In both cases I was asked*

during failed fertility treatment and for both there were more than
a few godparents. At one christening the other godmother literally
wouldn't let me hold the baby when I asked if I could; I don't know
if this was due to some kind of unspoken hierarchy of godmothers
or if she thought I'd drop the baby since I wasn't a mum!

Mandy: 44, Single, UK

When one of my nieces was sixteen, she asked me why, 'If nobody likes feminists, why are *you* one?' This started a fascinating conversation which continued on Facebook as I directed her towards various age-appropriate resources that I felt might help to counter the cultural rubbishing of women's power she'd been exposed to. I'm pretty sure this isn't a conversation she would have had with her mother.

Lesbians

In a 2012 article by comedian Chloe Hilliard titled 'I'm Not a Lesbian, I'm Just Childless', Hilliard writes:

> I'm thirty-one years old, black and childless. Coming from an African-American family with strong southern roots, that means either I can't have kids or I'm a lesbian.[104]

Newsflash! First and foremost, lesbians are actually *women*. Whoa, hold onto your hats, folks! They have the same fertility window as heterosexual women, the same infertility issues and, for those of them who hope to be mothers, the same issues in finding the 'right' relationship to bring a family into. Some of them are also with partners who already have children from earlier relationships and so many of them face the childless-by-relationship issue too.

Being a single childless woman doesn't mean you're a lesbian; it's wanting to partner with a woman you love passionately that does.

Sometimes, calling a childless woman a lesbian is a way of insulting her, of suggesting that she's either too 'strident' (i.e. has a mind of her own) or too ugly to 'get a man', because that's what conservative culture still thinks of lesbians – that they're not 'real women'. Whilst the LGBT community has been steadily becoming more visible for years now, the journey for childless/childfree women has only just begun. We have a lot to learn from them, in particular how they have reclaimed many of the words that used to be insults, as well as supporting each other and forming a tribe. And how they are prepared to call out prejudice when they see it and refuse to be shamed into silence by the insults directed at them.

Unlike heterosexual women, people don't seem to automatically jump to the conclusion that lesbian women already have children or must want to have children soon. The hidden prejudice here is that by *not* being heterosexual, lesbian women aren't real women (aren't you getting tired of all the ways we can somehow not be real women?!) and that therefore they're obviously not going to be maternal.

> *Being a lesbian woman, not many of my friends decide to become parents. Some have kids from prior relationships, some do go through the uphill struggle that is becoming a lesbian parent, some have even adopted. Those without kids understand the pain I went through ten years ago, to an extent, but really can't understand the yearning of a childless woman at times. Those with kids are just like any other woman with kids – somewhat oblivious.*
>
> Claude: 44, Single, UK

Whilst perhaps it might possibly be a relief *not* to get bombarded with the 'When are you going to have a baby?' or, 'How many kids have you got?' questions, in other ways, it's a double-negative discounting of lesbians as women. Not thinking of them as possible mothers is yet another way of 'othering' them from mainstream society.

Wicked Stepmothers

In fairy tales, the evil or wicked stepmother is a kind of witch who, by her very existence, seems to have stolen the place of the children's rightful mother and be in competition for their father's love. So of course she's going to want to get rid of them as soon as possible! In order to be truly evil (think of Snow White's stepmother) she also needs to be childless, so that she's one of those unnatural women to whom nature 'wisely' gave no children. If she was a mother herself, it would be harder to make her truly evil, as it would fight against the stereotype of mothers as good and selfless.

It's horrible to think that somewhere in the back of people's minds we could be viewed like this. The very idea of being seen as a threat to children, a type of 'child hater', is one of the most potent of all the shaming stereotypes that can be projected onto childless women; it's a double dose of shame: bad mother *and* childless woman.

This 'wickedness' is projected most strongly onto childfree women, who are considered to be unnatural in their active choice not to have children, although the reasons for their choices are often as complex as our reasons for becoming childless. Because it's quite common for people to presume that a childless woman has chosen her childlessness, we too often get tarred with the same ridiculous brush. However, even if others *do* know that we are involuntarily childless, the taboo nature of our situation carries *such* weight that we too may subconsciously be considered unnatural and therefore, in some subtle way, touched by evil, by wickedness. The fears that attach to childlessness are deep in human history, and not always conscious. They can carry a very big charge ...

As more than one childless woman has told me, people have suggested to them that obviously they were not 'fit' to be mothers in some way and that God knew that! And some of those comments have come from members of the clergy or other organised religions.

To be a stepmother is, in some sense, to accept that you are the wrong woman in the wrong place at the wrong time for your partner's children. When you are also childless yourself (not always by choice

– sometimes your partner doesn't want more children or it's just not possible for a whole host of reasons), being a stepmother is doubly hard. If you get very close to your stepchildren you might be accused of trying to usurp their mother's role, and if the relationship with them is stormy, you may well hear that it's likely your fault because, as you're not a mother, you don't know what you're doing. The fact that the relationship with your partner's children is difficult because everyone has been placed in a less than ideal position doesn't often seem to be acknowledged.

From the childless stepmothers who've shared their experiences in the Gateway Women online community, I can see how they're often made to feel that they don't have a voice in the family situation, even though they often do a good deal of the day-to-day parenting.

Witches

The fear of the childless woman has deep roots in our culture. If you think of both modern and ancient fairy tales, whether it's the evil scheming of Snow White's stepmother or the self-obsession, vanity and insanity of Cruella de Vil in *101 Dalmatians*, older childless women are *never* the heroines; things rarely end well for them.

> *I often feel like I am characterised as a 'witch' if I am not the way others want me to be. So either you are obedient or you're a witch. How can any self-respecting adult female live with that?*
>
> Margot: 67, Married, USA

This cultural prejudice against older childless women goes back to a time when women's knowledge as healers, herbalists and midwives became feared by the Church, as it was the continuation of ancient pagan knowledge from a pre-Christian era. In a time when having a large family was the only way to ensure that you had enough labour for your land and that you would be taken care of in old age, when childbirth was perilous and infant mortality high (as is still the case in the developing world), local healers had enormous prestige for their skill in helping mothers and children survive. They were also slightly feared, as they were 'apart' (different) from other women.

Often living without a family and on the edge of villages, they were consulted by local leaders for their wisdom. It is thought that such healers and midwives had knowledge of herbs to prevent pregnancies and ease deliveries, as well as to promote fertility or cause a miscarriage. The power invested in these 'wise women' was revered and feared by men and their knowledge was passed on orally. In a time before literacy, experienced older people were the libraries of their time, and valued and respected for this.

> *I've decided to embrace my 'inner witch' stereotype. My little black cat (Mojo!) is the perfect 'familiar'. Listen, women through the centuries have been punished (literally burned or drowned!) for daring to step outside what society seems to expect, i.e. if a woman isn't appended to a man or a child, she is crazy or dangerous in some way! That's fine with me. I prefer to think of all the powerful, beautiful aspects, i.e. being liberated, free, independent, creative, fun. So not all bad!*
>
> Maxime: 43, In a Relationship, UK

During the Renaissance in Europe, traditional women healers' knowledge began to be seen increasingly as being in conflict with the teachings and authority of the Church. Wise women and midwives were branded as 'witches' and hunted down and killed. It is estimated that 200,000 witches were accused and 100,000 were executed – either burned alive or drowned – during the witch hunts of the seventeenth century, although accurate records are difficult to find.[105] It was a female holocaust, eradicating both ancient knowledge and putting a fear of feminine power and mystery at the very centre of modern patriarchy and culture.

From the eradication of powerful women (and goddesses) from the Bible, including the writings that showed that the Hebrew god Yahweh had a wife and consort called Asherah,[106] through to the destruction of pagan fertility goddesses by the spread of Christianity and the burning of witches, feminine power and mystery have been shamed into silence and erased from history. Only youth and motherhood have retained any prestige as they serve to protect male interests. We have lived for so long under patriarchy (literally 'the rule of the father') that it seems normal to live like this, but it's a worn-out system.

A much more egalitarian way of viewing both men and women is needed. A system which shames, sidelines and ignores one in five women from their forties onwards and therefore keeps many of them at the margin of society, feeling unable to contribute in productive ways, is not just unfair, it's unsustainable and counter-productive to the development of our culture.

Change takes time, and courage. There is an expression, 'courage in a woman is often mistaken for insanity', which says it all really! We can stay quiet and out of sight (and miserable) or make a noise and risk being thought nuts. Having tried the former and almost disappeared with sadness, I now choose the latter.

Choose Your Own Label

Once you start using the internet to connect with other women without children, you discover that there are a lot of terms and labels to describe us.

Childless, childfree, CBC (childless-by-choice), CNBC (childless-not-by-choice), DINKS (double-income-no-kids), PANKS (professional-aunt-no-kids), GINKS (green-inclinations-no-kids), unparents, childful, nullipara, notmoms, barren, sterile, infertile, nomos . . .

I quite like the term 'solo'. It's gender neutral and I think has a
more positive connotation for single women without children.

Eimear: 44, Single, Ireland

I came up with the term 'nomo' because I wanted one that didn't include the word 'child', could be applied to any woman without children and sounded a bit groovy. It's an abbreviation of 'not-mother', or 'non-mother', and can be used for both childless and childfree women, but, like all terms, it will find its own way in the world and may stick or not. At first, I didn't think about it being used for *all* women without children, but journalists have picked up on it that way and that's how it's been used in the media.[107] Time will tell.

> *I like 'nomo' the best. Childless is good also. The more unapologetic the better.*
>
> Margot: 67, Married, USA

Some of us dislike the term 'nomo' and prefer to use 'Gateway Woman' (which I like, of course!). And many childless women disagree strongly with the notion of having a label at all.

In my blog 'The Gateway Women Manifesto: Are Childless Women the New Suffragettes?' I wrote:

> Yes, I know it's annoying that we need a label at all . . . Interestingly, the suffragettes thought so too – the term was coined by that famously 'women-friendly' newspaper the *Daily Mail* to ridicule members of the Women's Social and Political Union. Which they then reclaimed and made their own. No one uses the term suffragette anymore. Why? Because their work is done and we accept that women have as much right to vote as men. So we don't need the label anymore.[108]

As childless women, we are outsiders in mainstream culture. I understand the women who don't want a label apart from 'woman'. But sometimes we need to give up a little bit of our individuality to create some solidarity; to show how many we are and what we're really like. Finding a positive label to define us is difficult because most of us don't want to be labelled at all. Yet I believe we need one in order to come together as a tribe, and then together to outgrow it.

If you don't want a label, I can completely get that. I don't really want one either! But consider this: perhaps by *not* finding one that you feel OK about identifying with, you're actually participating in the silent shaming that perpetuates our outsider status? We've got nothing to be ashamed of. The fact is, others have given you a label and they use it when you're not listening – wouldn't you rather choose your own?

To name something is a powerful thing. It creates a reality. It owns it. Just as homosexual men and women have reclaimed 'gay', 'queer' and 'dyke' as terms that *they* define the meaning for, not others, child-less women who won't be silenced or shamed by how things have turned out for them now need a term to rally behind. When we find one that the vast majority of us feel comfortable with and proud of, we'll already be halfway to not needing it anymore. Although I agree that 'woman' and 'human' would be better, I just don't think we're quite there yet.

EXERCISE 5
Role Models

Step 1:

Get together a selection of popular mainstream women's magazines. It doesn't matter if they're not the sort of thing you normally read. Cut out any images or references you can find to childless or childfree women. Using the categories and stereotypes we've been looking at in this chapter, or any others that arise, see if you can sort them into groups of some kind.

Once you've done this think about the following questions:

- What sort of ratio can you find between positive and negative portrayals of women without children?

- How do you feel about yourself as a childless woman after this exercise?

Step 2:

Take a look at the Gateway Women role model gallery on Pinterest: bit.ly/gw-role-models. There are over 500 women here, both contemporary and historical, with their photos and their mini-biographies. Remember that these women do not represent all childless or childfree women, only the ones who have a public profile of some kind. It does not mean that you have to do something that merits a public profile just because you are childless – it just makes you more visible!

Once you've had a good look consider the following:

- How do you feel about yourself as a childless woman after this exercise?

- Do you have a sense now of how media representations of women without children affect you?

A few more questions to ponder:

- Is there a derogatory name, label or archetype for older childless women that you fear being applied to you?

- Is there an older, childless or childfree woman you admire in your family, community, workplace, or in the public eye? What is it about her that speaks to you? Can you think of a way to open a dialogue with her?

- How do you feel about childfree-by-choice women? Is there anything you think about them that you wouldn't want people to think about you? Are you perhaps prejudiced towards them in ways that you fear people are prejudiced against you? Can you see that it might not be true?

- What label do you choose for yourself? Even if you don't want one, you've already got one; it's just that others probably don't use it to your face. It might be 'that sad woman who couldn't have kids and never got over it', or 'that witch from accounts'. Wouldn't you rather people started using a label you've chosen for yourself?

Reflections on Chapter 5

In this chapter we've explored how childless women are perceived in our culture and, in turn, how we perceive ourselves. Sometimes, beginning to lift the lid on this stuff can be quite explosive, so if you've found yourself getting a bit hot under the collar over the last week, that's quite normal.

Exploring some of the things we deal with in casual conversation, at family gatherings, with our parents and siblings and at work may begin to bring into focus for you how childless women face outdated and prejudicial views in so many different areas of our lives. You may be feeling that you're ready to 'go into battle' on behalf of yourself and your childless sisters, but hold your horses just for now! Sometimes it feels easier to get angry on behalf of others than ourselves, but until we've felt and understood our own emotions, and analysed and reality-tested our own conditioning and assumptions, it's best not to take them on the rampage. A great way to let off steam (and it's excellent grief work too) is to join a private online community for childless women and share your thoughts and feelings with others who will be prepared to enter into the debate with you without trying to close you down as 'bitter' or 'selfish' (two of the classic ways to silence an angry childless or childfree woman).

Beginning to explore some of the stereotypes that have settled on childless women can be pretty shocking. As we begin to realise how the ways in which we are viewed (and perhaps have viewed ourselves) may have contributed to our own unhappiness, we might be quite shocked and even feel quite foolish. It's important not to shame ourselves for this – we've done quite enough of that already. Realising how such views may have controlled our choices and beliefs in the past can be quite sad, but hopefully you will be inspired to continue your own education in these areas and decide what you want to think and believe about them. You'll find lots of resources and books in the Appendix.

Something to look out for is that you may begin to notice more the language that others use, and you might see changes in the language you use yourself. Also, you may begin to reflect on how other stigmatised or marginalised groups might feel about the way that they are spoken to, or about. Beginning to free our minds from such powerful conditioning is a gradual, exciting and sometimes painful process. It will take a while, maybe even a lifetime. You don't need to do it all right now ...

If you did the 'Role Models' exercise, you may have found yourself astonished by how narrow and negative the view is that the media (which is the amplifier of our culture) has of childless women. I hope that discovering the role model gallery showed you that the way the media represents us is far from any kind of 'truth' ...

Now you are beginning to see the world around you more clearly you can make some different choices, which will bring with them sometimes unwelcome, but ultimately liberating, responsibilities. As Eleanor Roosevelt famously said, 'No one can insult you without your permission.' A big part of getting your mojo back as a childless woman is to reclaim your power and identity as a woman who matters. If others don't agree, that's not our problem!

We only change when the

PAIN

of

CHANGING

*becomes
less painful than
the pain of*

NOT

changing.

CHAPTER 6

Who Moved My Mojo?

Dusting Off Your Dancing Shoes

After all the years of hoping, presuming, trying, crying, grieving, raging and coping with the whole damn 'baby thing', you probably wouldn't recognise your mojo if it came up to you and asked you to dance! And even then, you'd probably refuse. *Dance? You must be out of your mind ... I don't do* that *anymore!*

You may wonder if, after all you've been through, you actually *want* to find your mojo again. Sounds exhausting just thinking about it, doesn't it? Let alone actually doing something about it ... You feel sluggish, worn out and vague. You stay busy, *too busy*, at work, but at home you can't be bothered to do much at all. You're behind with all your life admin and surrounded by half-painted walls, unfinished projects and piles of books you can't quite get around to reading. You don't really have a social life anymore, which is quite a relief as you'd be embarrassed for anyone to see how you really live these days ...

It doesn't feel like a promising place from which to start anything, does it?

I used to think, 'must keep going', 'must be strong', 'it's nothing that should be making me feel bad'. But then I reached a point where I'd had enough; I reached out for help and took a few

*months off work. I felt empty, had no energy to do anything; the
housework and garden were ignored and I didn't care what didn't
get done. I stopped looking after myself, ate badly, drank too much,
and couldn't be bothered to do my hair or make-up. I just wanted to sleep and ignore everything. I think it was my body finally
saying to me, 'Enough!!!! You need to stop and deal with this and
heal,' so it shut down ...*

Delia: 48, Living with Partner, UK

After all, isn't this whole mojo thing a bit fanciful? Another bit of
new age mumbo-jumbo to get your hopes up, only to leave you one
book heavier and back where you started? Why bother?

Well, you always have the option to stay exactly where you are.

And in fact, you may *need* to stay there until you *can't* stay there
any more. In my own experience, change isn't something any of us
undertakes because it seems like a good idea. Well, not change that
sticks anyway. Because it appears that we only change when the pain of
not changing becomes more painful than the pain of changing.

*I've read a lot of self-help books in regard to dating and found
most of them useless. The books on childlessness that were most
helpful to me (including yours) were the ones that made me feel
less alone. My fears for myself if I didn't change were that I'd
spend my entire life feeling bitter, sad, and cheated.*

Sarah: 45, Single, USA

Change is not something we find easy because change is something
our ego sees as a risk factor and being risk-averse is a good biological
survival strategy. However, we need our ego, no matter how much of
a rough ride it gets in a lot of self-help literature; without it we'd be
unable to function in the world and would have to be locked up for our

own and others' safety. Our ego is a filtering and organising system that works out which parts of the endless stream of data coming our way are relevant and which aren't; what's a threat to us and what's not; who we are, and who we aren't. Its function is to make sense of randomness – to sift and filter all the information coming from our senses and create a comprehensible version of reality that keeps us safe and meets our needs. As far as the ego is concerned, any non-essential randomness (i.e. chosen change) is to be avoided as it increases risk.

The ego is also the part of our consciousness that creates our identity and gives us a sense of who we are compared to other people. It's always in flux, always assessing new data and accepting or rejecting the information as it fits with our prevailing idea *at the time* of who we are and what's important to us. Do you remember how it was when you longed to be pregnant and all you could see were pregnant women everywhere? That was your ego highlighting what was important to you at the time. It wasn't that fate had decided to put more pregnant women in your path just to break your heart a little bit more, even though it may have felt like it at the time.

Although it's beyond the scope of this book to explore the nature of the ego in depth, it's relevant here because realising that the idea of having a fixed identity, a 'me' who never changes, is actually an *illusion* can help to allay some of our fears that transitioning into a new Plan B identity isn't possible. You've already had many different 'identities' in your life so far. If you think about it, isn't your sense of 'yourself' today different from what it was when you were a child or a young woman? And yet, at the time, wouldn't you have said that those identities were absolutely 'you'? That's how the ego works: it presents a snapshot in time as something unchanging, but it's not the case. It's a mind trick, a technique our consciousness has evolved to help us cope with the ever-changing nature of reality.

One of the reasons that losing something or someone we consider vital to our sense of self is so painful is that the ego experiences it as an attack on our own identity, on our sense of who we think we are. I hope this helps you to understand why losing the potential identity of 'mother' can be so very hard to cope with. As so many of us know, you don't have to actually *be* a mother in order to have a huge part of our identity invested in the goal or role of motherhood.

The grieving process, like falling in love, involves a shift in our identity. We are never the same person again after loving someone or losing someone.

When we fall in love, our brain is flooded with chemicals that pretty much keep the ego too drunk to notice the radical structural renovations it's undertaking. With grief, denial is the mechanism that keeps the show on the road until your ego is ready to begin the shift to this new identity.

However, during the process of grieving (which is an active process, rather than the passive 'stuckness' of grief) there is a fluidity to our sense of self which offers us the chance to reconsider whether being fixated on our identity serves us in the long run. It's a transformational time, an opportunity to build a relationship with the 'witnessing' part of us that runs much deeper than our ego – the core part of our consciousness from which our ego developed. This is what mindfulness and meditation practices are for, but you don't need to meditate to take this first step; it's enough to start to wonder 'who' it is who is able to think about things like 'mind', 'identity' and 'ego'. Learning to notice this calm and more spacious part of ourselves can be the beginning of developing a more flexible approach to life, making the twists and turns of fate much easier to bear.

These days, I like to imagine myself as a tree with well-nourished roots. When storms come, as they always do, these days I bend with the wind. I try not to resist the wind, pretend it's not there, yell at it, get depressed by it or feel outraged because I don't deserve it. It's just wind and I bend. Sometimes, if I'm feeling a bit brittle and resistant – *Not fair! Not now! Not my turn! Not mine!* – I might snap a few branches here and there, but more and more frequently I bend as the storm passes through me and straighten myself back up afterwards. There was a time when I used to joke that the universe had put a sign on my back that read 'kick me' but I don't take life so personally any more. It just is what it is. Except on the days when I don't. I'm not special or different to anyone else; I'm like you, like all of us, a work in progress.

Your ego, your psyche, will change when it has to, when you're ready, and not a moment sooner. It might be that by reading this book you are laying the ground for change at a later date, or it might be that something in this book provides the catalyst you need to start changing. You may have already started.

Trust yourself. Yes, *you*, really. If you're not ready to make any changes yet, don't give yourself a hard time about it. It's not going to help and it won't speed things up. Your timing is just that: *your* timing. You can feed and water a plant and place it in the sun, but you can't make it grow any quicker than it grows.

Creating a Life of Meaning

In 1946, Viktor Frankl, a Viennese psychiatrist interned by the Nazis in various concentration camps, wrote a short memoir describing his experiences and outlining what was to become 'logotherapy' – a form of existential psychotherapy which focuses on finding a reason to live. At the time of his death in 1997, *Man's Search for Meaning* had been translated into twenty-four languages and had sold over ten million copies.[109]

This short book, which can be read in an afternoon, is absolutely life changing. It's about the power of the human spirit to survive, and even flourish, when every conceivable human right, need and dignity has been taken away. It's about the choice we all have, as human beings, in *any* situation, to choose how we are going to feel about it; to decide what meaning we are going to give it. In the book, Frankl quotes the philosopher Nietzsche: 'He who has a why to live can endure almost any how.' Make that a 'she'. Because without a 'why', even the most luxurious and comfortable existence can be a daily torment. You can count your blessings till the cows come home, but without a reason, a purpose for living, living itself can become a chore. I know that you know what I mean. A chore.

> *I've always felt the need to do work that means something to me, but I do get bored with my projects and jobs after some time. I thought having a child would always keep me on my toes, and I had hoped that would give my life meaning, at least for the next fifteen to twenty years. Remaining childless definitely sent me into an existential crisis. But I always felt that I would learn something from it. I don't know if there's a point to this existence, but I do know that humans make meaning, so you can always create your own meaningful life. And it doesn't have to be fixed. But you do need to learn how to deal with disappointment when meaning crumbles, and trust the process of creating new meaning. I don't think my life is ever meaningless, but sometimes I don't see it – life can look pretty bleak at those times … But there is always the upswing where life is brilliant again.*
>
> Marjon: 43, Engaged, The Netherlands

It is perhaps only other childless women who can understand the depth of existential despair that many of us experience, and which leaves us wondering if we have the courage to face the rest of our lives feeling like this. It is a dark night of the soul of such profundity that, if faced and transcended, creates a depth of psychological maturity and compassion in us that very few other adults around us can match. We have looked our death-in-life in the face and survived it. We live with ghosts that no one but us ever knew.

Finding a way to create a life of meaning from a place of existential bleakness is an act of great moral courage, and absolutely essential if we are to enjoy, rather than merely endure, the rest of our life.

Frankl's book, and the school of existential psychotherapy that he founded, shows that finding the meaning of life is a unique journey for each of us. No one has the answer for you, no one can tell you what your meaning is. And most of us don't even know what it is until we find it. Finding your meaning is like falling in love: you know it when it happens.

> *I'm absolutely seeking a life of meaning now! All of this grief and loss for a life without meaning? No way! We have all paid dearly with our heartbreaks; it's time to party!*
>
> Kyla: 43, Married, USA

As well as being a gift to ourselves, finding and creating a life of meaning is a gift to those around us and to the wider world. Hopefully we've all met people whose lives are shaped in such a way that allows them to express what's most important to them. They shine in a way that others don't, and they give courage and hope to all they meet. We live in cynical times, but when we meet someone who has learned how to make their soul sing, ours sings too.

We have a choice.

When we are ready, we can create our new life around something that makes us feel alive in the way that we were convinced *only* having a child could. Or we can flounder for years, never really living, just existing.

> *Two and a half years after starting my grief work, 'creating a life of meaning' seems to be the most important and exciting part of my every breathing moment as the blinkers have been lifted! (Now that's not something I would have written three years ago). It does seem like a big project, but it's such an empowering new stage of my life. I am just chipping away at my life to achieve my Plan B.*
>
> Laura: 47, Single, UK

You'll know when you're ready to make this transition and there's no shame in taking your time. It takes as long as it takes and shortcuts don't work – I have the mileage on the clock to prove it! Grieving is an exhausting process and change requires energy. You may need some more time to top up your reserves.

Far from planning this, if your experience is anything like mine, you'll realise in retrospect that you've already taken the first step. This is not something you can put on a to-do list or schedule – just as you cannot schedule falling in love. But what you *can* do is your groundwork, so that when that moment comes, you're ready. And that's what this book is for.

Whatever Happened to 'Desperately Seeking Susan'?

If I cast my mind back to what I was like in my early twenties, I think I was probably rather scary. Very tall, dramatically dressed and with a bravado mask of bullish confidence that hid my utter cluelessness about who I was. An adult in physical form only. My role model was the character Madonna played in *Desperately Seeking Susan*, a film that came out in 1985 when I was turning twenty-one. I went to the cinema over and over again (this was before video) to see the film, so stunned was I by this radically new idea of how to be a woman. Susan/Madonna was totally unlike anything else I'd seen up until that point in my life. She was ballsy, independent, fearless and sexy and seemed to be running her life just the way *she* wanted it.

After a childhood where I'd learned that your happiness as a woman was largely dictated by the behaviour of the men in your life, Susan's complete disregard for men's opinions, her offhand treatment of their affection and her disregard for the rules of society intoxicated me. Now, although I couldn't sing and had no desire to be a pop star, I was thrilled and inspired by Susan as she busted her way out of what women were 'allowed' to do, think or say and, encouraged and inspired by that, I took life head on, artfully ripped fishnet tights and all!

Fast-forward around twenty years to my late thirties and I'd been through the tumble dryer of life: I'd seen bad things happen to good people; I'd witnessed the love of my life succumbing to a heartbreaking drink and drug addiction, and spent my thirties suffering from unexplained infertility and watching our business, home and marriage be consumed by my husband's addictions (and my co-dependency). I ended up on the floor, literally and metaphorically, a nervous wreck at thirty-seven.

Picking myself up from that, fuelled by babymania and with total confidence (or rather in complete denial) that at the age of forty, and after eleven years of 'unexplained infertility', I'd be remarried and a mother (via IVF) in a couple of years, I propelled myself into the (then) brave new world of online dating. And with babymania as the fuel in my rocket-propelled dating engine, I made some very bizarre decisions with regard to my career, finances and relationships over the next few years.

Coming out of the tunnel of denial at forty-four and a half (the only people other than children under ten who count their years in halves are women running out of time to conceive), I had no idea who I was anymore. If someone had said to me at that point that what I needed to do was to 'construct a new identity around a life of meaning', I think I would have looked at them, understood the words, but wouldn't have had a clue what they were talking about.

But one thing I absolutely knew for sure was that what had excited me in my twenties wasn't going to do it for me anymore – for goodness' sake, even Madonna had married an Englishman and taken up hunting! However, I seriously doubted if I had the energy to get excited about anything ever again. I'd try reading books and lose interest after about fifty pages; I'd go to art galleries or museums and all I could think about was getting to the cake shop. I felt about a thousand years old and bored with both life and myself – and dangerously uninspired.

Dreams? Goals? Ambitions? Practically none left. I was a spent force, an empty vessel. An ageing and defective woman, alone in her forties, broke physically, financially, emotionally and spiritually.

But gradually I began to realise that what had happened is not that I didn't have any dreams anymore, but that I'd <u>neglected</u> them for so long that I'd forgotten <u>how</u> to have them.

It took a great deal of courage to start imagining a future again because deep down I was terrified of dreaming again: the dream of marriage and family had cost me so dear, it seemed too risky to dare to dream of *anything*, ever again. I genuinely thought that another disappointment, another failure, would finish me off completely, so it seemed safer not to even try.

I felt stuck, with no idea how to move forward. And so I started where I always start, with my first love, writing. For a couple of years, I just kept journals, but I was bored with the sound of my voice on paper, bored to tears of the inside of my head. So then I tried blogging and it seemed that the notion that I was potentially writing for someone other than myself, even just *one* reader, helped me to reconnect with my inner storyteller – the mystical, philosophical and cheeky little girl I'd once been and who I felt I'd lost. She was still in there, waiting for me.

I discovered that even though I felt ancient and almost suffocated by grief-related depression, my capacity to dream had not been completely extinguished. It may have only been a whisper of a flame, but my pilot light was still on.

And so is yours. Because you wouldn't still be reading if it weren't . . .

Russian Dolls

Grab a pile of Post-it notes or small pieces of paper. Use them to write down individual words or phrases that come to mind in response to this exercise.

Imagine yourself as if you were a series of Russian dolls, with the biggest doll being the 'you' you are today, and the smallest doll being the 'you' you were when you were born. Each and every 'you' lives on as a part of you today, along with her hopes and dreams.

Although right now it may feel that the hopeful dreamer in you is well and truly vanquished, I'd like to suggest that she's still in there somewhere. In fact, there's proof: take a moment to recall what it's like when you smell something that instantly transports you back to a childhood memory. In that moment, you *are* that age again, with all its rich, vivid aliveness.

Here are three questions to help you connect with three of your Russian dolls – you at three different stages of your girlhood:

- Around the age of five (or just starting your first school)

- Around the age of ten (or just before puberty)

- Around the age of fifteen (or just becoming a young woman)

Write the answers to each of the following questions separately. The prompts below don't necessarily *all* have to be answered – they're just ways to remind you of the kinds of things you may (or may not) have been doing at each age. You might find that it jogs your memory and completely different things come up.

Question 1: What did you love doing when you were a young girl?
Sit on the floor to answer these, cross-legged or in any position that's

comfortable. Try to 'see' the world from the height you were when you were around the age of five or six.

1. What did you want to be or do when you grew up?

2. Did you like to play in nature or perhaps stay indoors alone or with friends?

3. Did you like building things with Lego? What did you build?

4. Did you like painting and drawing? What did you paint or draw?

5. Were you an avid reader, writer or storyteller? What kinds of books or stories?

6. Were you physically very competent – riding a bike and climbing trees younger than most – or perhaps more timid, needing encouragement to try new things?

7. Did you take every chance to be in the kitchen learning to cook? What were your favourite things to cook?

8. Were you described as a 'tomboy', 'bookworm' or 'princess', or something else like that?

9. Did you lie on your back and gaze at the clouds and think about the nature of reality?

10. Did you enjoy playing with dolls or did you perhaps find them a bit silly?

11. Did you grow things in your garden? What did you grow?

12. Did you love dressing up in your mother's clothes and shoes and putting on make-up?

Question 2: What did you love doing just before puberty?
Lie on your stomach, lean against the wall, curl up in an armchair – whatever position you recall being your 'thinking' position when you were around ten or eleven (or before puberty started).

1. Did you like making things with your hands? What kinds of things?

2. Did you like 'homemaking' hobbies like quilting, sewing, cooking, etc.?

3. Were you in the Girl Guides or Girl Scouts? What did you like about it?

4. Did you run wild in nature alone, or with your friends?

5. Were you a daredevil or more bookish?

6. Did you enjoy school? Did you find it limited or bored you in some way? If there was something you wanted to be doing more than school, what was it?

7. Did you read teenage magazines and want to be grown up?

8. Did you think about your future family and have someone you talked about as being the person you were going to marry and have children with one day?

9. Did you read fantasy stories? What did you dream of being – a witch, a princess, a talking horse, an angel, an amazon, a mermaid, an adventurer, an avenger ... ?

10. Were you in a gang? What was your role?

11. What was your role in your family by this time? The 'difficult' one, the 'bookish' one, the 'caring' one, the 'problem' one, the 'good girl' ... ?

12. Did you have something you wanted to do or be when you grew up? Was there someone you looked up to or idolised? Who were they?

Question 3: What did you enjoy (or not) about school?

Sit at a desk in a hard chair. Try to sit in the position that feels like the one you would have been in at school when you were around the age of fifteen.

1. Was there a subject that you loved but weren't very good at so you dropped it? What was it?

2. Was there a subject that you took extra care with when you did your homework? What was it?

3. Was there a teacher that you remember as particularly inspiring?

What subject did they teach? What was it about them that captivated you?

4. Did you hate lessons, but love a different aspect of school such as sport, socialising, music, debating, chess, amateur dramatics, gossip ... ?

5. Was there an out-of-school activity you were more inspired by than school activities, such as a book club, sports club, drama club, Girl Guides ... ?

6. What 'crowd' did you hang around with? Did you have a 'role' in that crowd?

7. If you preferred being on you own, do you think there was something 'different' about you? Were you OK with that?

8. Were you a natural leader, a bit of a rebel or perhaps a peacemaker?

9. Did you wish there were subjects you could study that weren't available at your school, or that 'girls' didn't do?

10. If you hated school and played truant a lot, do you know what it was about school that you hated? What did you do when you weren't in school?

11. Did you long for the holidays or were you counting the days to the return to school?

12. If you could have your schooldays over again, would you do anything differently?

Take a look at the answers to all three questions at the same time. If they're on Post-it notes or pieces of paper, see if you can start putting answers or ideas together that seem to have similarities.

- Can you see any themes emerging?
- How do you feel when you think about those themes?
- Can you feel a tickle of joy in your gut when you think about one or some of them?

- Notice if you feel fear or any other strong emotion about any of them – this may be a clue that you are attracted to it, but that you may have learned to be nervous of excitement or joy.

Taking Little Steps

It's important to pay attention to anything that gives you a tingle of joy or even remembered joy. Human beings are meaning-making beings, and one of the clues that lead us towards our meaning is joy. When we were children we naturally gravitated towards those things that brought us joy – we found them meaningful, even if no one else agreed with us. As adults many of us have lost that simple connection to meaning, buried under 'shoulds' and 'musts', until we find it hard to know what moves us anymore. We also make judgements and criticisms of ourselves such as, 'It's ridiculous for a grown woman to enjoy ...' (insert whatever thing you just thought of!).

When I was a young girl, I used to look at grown-ups and think, *They've got as much pocket money as they want, they can go to bed when they want, they can read what they want, they can eat what they want ... so why are they all so miserable?* It's amusing, but it's also something that we forget as adults – we're much more in charge of our happiness than we realise ...

I've had such a desire to revisit those activities that I loved from my childhood – horse-riding lessons, spending time with animals, swimming in rivers, feeling free, not wearing a watch. I have tried to incorporate these desires as they come up into my actual reality (ha ha!) and have found that they are exactly what I need – they bring me a sense of peace and a connection with the deeper me, the me before trauma and loss, the real me.

Sally: 39, Married, Canada

The grief of childlessness can rob us of our capacity to take joy in the things we used to like. We can be stuck in unprocessed grief for so long that it begins to feel like a permanent character change. Add to this the hormonal changes of menopause (more on that in Chapter 8) and you can end up in a joyless funk that lasts for years.

Whilst you can't *force* yourself to enjoy life's pleasures again if you're still processing your grief, what you *can* do is to start doing the work to uncover your joy. As we learned earlier, grief is a spiral – not a series of linear steps – and it may be that you can cope with a small dose of joy now, and work up to a life full of joy as the loving energy of grief heals you and prepares you to open up to the world again.

> *At first, thinking about 'meaning' did feel like a big and scary project, but these days I'm far more relaxed about letting it unfold. The biggest step was letting go of the ideas I had held onto with a vice-like grip about how my life was supposed to be (husband, house, children) and being open to what might still be. I am curious about that and feel excited about the future again.*
>
> Natasha: 53, Single, UK

Sometimes, we have to meet life halfway. Show that we're willing to change and then allow ourselves to be changed. You just have to take that first tiny step.

Forget your to-do lists and all the 'grown-up' things you need to get done before you can even <u>consider</u> doing something 'just for fun'. On the day you die, there will still be things left to do on your to-do list.

By gently opening your heart to joy again now, you stand a chance of being a woman who lived a life that fed her soul, rather than someone who put off her joy in order to get her chores done.

EXERCISE 7

Little Steps Towards Meaning

Take a look at some of the ideas that the 'Russian Dolls' exercise brought up for you — some of the things that made you feel that tickle of joy (or fear). Is there a way that you could bring a little bit of this into your life over the next week? Nothing huge, but something that takes you towards joy or deep satisfaction.

If that exercise didn't bring up anything for you, perhaps there's something you've been wondering about exploring for a while but haven't yet stepped towards?

It might be baking a cake or enquiring about going back to study a subject you once loved. It could be getting back in touch with an old friend or getting your bike out of the garage. Maybe it's buying a new sketchbook and doing a drawing for yourself, or perhaps switching off the TV and being with the silence in your life.

Make it as easy to do as possible and commit to it. Nothing elaborate. The first little step only.

Expect and prepare for the possibility of a surprising amount of resistance to following this through! If you don't manage to do it in the next week, write down all the reasons you came up with as to why you couldn't do it and please don't feel ashamed. This tiny step is a BIG challenge to your ego and it may not let you get away with it first time. Whatever you do or don't do, it's not failure; it's feedback.

Reflections on Chapter 6

In this chapter we've started to explore the reasons behind why creating a life of meaning for ourselves as childless women isn't some kind of self-indulgent way to fill the time, but is actually a way to save our lives. And why that can be really hard work, even though it's what we crave with all our hearts.

How was it for you to see that perhaps your resistance to change is not some kind of personal character failure, but something that is hard-wired into human nature – one of your survival mechanisms, no less? Change is hard for everyone – once you knew that, did you start to realise that it might be possible to let go of your identity as an unhappily childless woman? Or did you find that rather challenging? Or maybe a bit of both?

Beginning to think about creating a life of meaning can feel quite overwhelming at times. And motherhood may seem as if it is the existential get-out-of-jail-free card, but it doesn't always work and, even if it does, it doesn't last. Children grow up and leave home and what comes after that is rarely the fantasy that commercials peddle.

If you did the 'Russian Dolls' exercise, what came up for you? Some women find that they have very few memories of their childhoods. If that was the case for you, perhaps you chose to focus on a different time in your life? If you were able to imagine your younger versions of yourself, how was that for you? In my experience and in my workshops, when we excavate our past like this, it can bring up a mixture of both hope and sadness. Sadness is part of adjusting to loss and deserves to be acknowledged too.

If you did the 'Little Steps Towards Meaning' exercise, how did it feel to open that tiny little window in your soul and let in some fresh air? Did it give you just the teensiest bit of hope that perhaps, in time, you might be able to feel good about your life again? Or did that taste of happiness scare you, by reminding you how very far you've gone from your true self? Did it perhaps make you sad to realise how hard it is, right now, to give yourself a treat and do something that you enjoy? And if you tried to do the exercise but found that, despite your best intentions, you found a whole host of reasons not to follow through with it, perhaps that's given you some insight into what a good job your ego does in protecting you from change! Hopefully you've now got some really useful feedback to enable you to recalibrate and try again. It might be that you made your Little Step too 'worthy', too 'sensible' or too 'ambitious' – and it was hard to find the impetus to do it. There again, you may have found yourself sneering at it as too 'childish' or 'frivolous' for a grown-up woman with 'things to do' ... When you're ready, have another go at taking a Little Step – there's no rush. And don't bother giving yourself a hard time for not doing it – it won't get you there any faster. In fact, it'll slow you down and even shut you down.

All of these feelings, and others, are quite normal. It's usually the meaning, the 'story' we attach to our feelings, that causes the problem. Imagine for a moment that you'd been sitting in a darkened room for some time, longing for daylight. When it came, that longed-for sun on your face would be too bright, perhaps even painful. But it wouldn't mean that you'd want to go back into the dark again. You'd squint, and wait for your eyes to adjust. It's the same for us as we move towards our Plan B.

When our
broken dreams
have cost us so dear,
dreaming
A NEW DREAM
takes great
COURAGE.

CHAPTER 7

Letting Go of Your Burned-out Dreams

The Shadow Life

When I knew for sure that I was never going to have a biological child of my own I became acutely aware that for many years I'd been living two lives: one in which I was hoping for a baby and making the best of things till then, the other in which I had succeeded and had become a mother.

I call the life I wasn't living my 'shadow life'. I was, in fact, a 'shadow mother'.

At no point in that time (a fifteen-year stretch no less) did I fully and completely embrace the life I was *actually* living – that of a childless woman. I was always in transition to the next stage when my *real* life would begin. As a result my reality often felt like a poor fit, but I ascribed my unhappiness and dissatisfaction to the fact that I *wasn't a mother*, rather than it being the very *wanting to be a mother* that was making me miserable. In Buddhism, it is said that the root of all human suffering is 'craving'. Recovering from the pain of childlessness, I came to understand that the root of my unhappiness wasn't that I didn't give birth to my longed-for child, but the *craving* I'd had for that child.

I don't doubt that I wanted a child and that I would have been delighted to have become a mother. However, I was totally unable to entertain the idea that I could be happy if that didn't work out.

Even thinking about it felt disloyal, as if it would make it less likely to happen.

Like so many of us I became so obsessed with having a child, over such a long period of time, that I stopped examining *why* I wanted this, or even whether I really did anymore. It feels terrible to write that, even now. It feels disloyal to myself, my dreams and the family I longed for. And it's precisely that irrational fear (i.e. denial) that prevented me from re-examining my dreams and options when I started dating again after my divorce. I was so familiar with being obsessed with becoming a mother that I went head first into looking for a new life partner who was willing to do IVF with me before time ran out. I reassessed everything else about my life, but I left my dream of becoming a mother untouched and unexamined.

Gripped by babymania, I made some truly awful decisions about relationships, career and finances. By being too afraid to hold my dream of motherhood up to the light in case I lost it, I kept myself in the dark about who I now was and what I wanted from the rest of my life. It actually didn't even occur to me to *consider* the possibility of a Plan B or the idea that a life without children might, in the end, suit me just fine. It honestly didn't enter my mind.

Letting go of the dream of motherhood was perhaps the single hardest thing I have ever done. It was wrenchingly painful and took years. The shadow life was more real for me than my real life. I was so consumed with the idea of finding a man and having a family that I held on long after I could have realistically conceived and in doing so neglected family, friends and myself. It diminished my real life enormously. It is still hard to look at that now, but I do so these days with self-compassion, not self-blame.

Natasha: 53, Single, UK

Because I never allowed myself to imagine that a life without children was possible, I never gave it any energy – which means that I never really put any energy into the life I was *actually* living. No wonder it was a mess. I starved my lived reality of life force and then I wondered why it felt like I was dying inside …

The Dark Side of Daydreams

I think of the 'shadow life' as the life you dreamed about while your 'real life' was happening, and to which you gave so much energy that it depleted the life you were actually living. I see it as the shadow of the life unlived. I'm not saying that dreaming about motherhood was wrong; it's perhaps just the *amount* of energy you invested in those daydreams that was unbalanced.

When your daydreams are sucking the life force out of your lived life, you've sprung a psychic leak!

Letting go of your shadow life means that first you have to bring it into the light of your awareness and take a good look at it. This can be quite scary because it's a bit like waking up and trying to put a dream into words and feeling the 'meaning' of your dream slip away. What felt magical becomes prosaic and you feel the loss. It seems safer to keep it all to yourself. Doing this will also probably bring more grief to the surface, but perhaps you might be ready to see that as more healing rather than as a signal to repress those thoughts, those feelings.

There are really no words to explain how difficult it was to work as a midwife while continually saying goodbye to my own babies through pregnancy loss, infertility and a million broken dreams. My shadow life was most definitely out of sync with my daily reality, and it was not until I was able to stop both versions and begin to consider something else entirely that I started to feel even remotely whole.

Sally: 39, Married, Canada

If in your shadow life as a mother you imagined a loving partner and playing in the garden with your children, whilst in your real life you were both single and living in an apartment with a window box full of dead plants, there's a kind of disconnect between these two that doesn't feel great. When you bring it into the light, it can stir up feelings of anger, bitterness, blame, depression and resentment. This is a natural part of grief, and letting go is what grief is all about.

> *I think the hardest thing for me is to let go of a dream of family since I had such a hostile one growing up. I think that when you have that hole, the longing for a family is especially hard to give up. I think the longing will always be with me. We all need accept-ance and that is what family often means.*
>
> Margot: 67, Married, USA

Hanging on to an old dream takes a lot of energy – energy that could be better used making a new, maybe even better life, come into being.

Letting go of daydreams is hard because, frankly, letting go of anything is hard ...

When I was still hopeful of having a child and completely in denial about the reality of my situation, I felt I couldn't change the movie in my personal dream cinema because, if I did, maybe I was being disloyal to my dreams of becoming a mother. I think at some deep level I under-stood that this dream was sucking the life out of me but I refused to allow it to evolve as my life took a different direction. The kind of self-reflective analysis I would apply to any other area of my life I withheld from this part. I was too scared to look closely because it felt like the 'dream' was all I had left. Letting go of my dream of motherhood felt like letting go of that very last part of me that *was* a mother. I fought it like hell. But once I was ready, it wasn't nearly as bad as I expected. Now, at night, I don't dream of babies anymore. Not flying babies, not being pregnant, not of a little girl holding my hand. I dream of other things, new things.

> *For a long time I had an image in my head about what being a mother would be like and almost feeling like it was 'the key to happiness'. Over time I now realise that it's society's expectation of us to get married, have a child and have another one, etc. I'm now very aware that there are no guarantees that having a child will bring us the ultimate fulfilment we desire; but the fact that the choice has been taken away takes time to adjust to.*
>
> Katie: 33, Married, UK

You can't force this stage because truly letting go of this dream is a major loss. We're losing our family. Only you'll know when you're ready to let go of the string and let this fantasy balloon float away ...

Getting to Know Your Shadow Life

Each of us who wanted to become a mother has our own themes and storylines in our shadow story, but here are some that you might recognise in yours.

The Happy Family Fantasy

For many of us, what we craved was not just a baby, but a family. We wanted to be part of something, to create something bigger than ourselves. Yes, we craved the unconditional love of an infant, but we also wanted a partner and siblings in the picture. We saw ourselves in the kitchen, at family gatherings. Perhaps you had a snapshot in your mind of a perfect little family, like the iconic families used by advertising to sell us stuff? But ask yourself this – weren't we perhaps being a little unreasonable expecting our family to turn out perfectly? Do you actually know any perfect families? Is your own family of origin perfect? Like all shadow life vignettes, there's nothing weird about this.

However, perhaps you might like to wonder if part of your longing for a perfect family was in some way driven by a need to right the wrongs of your own childhood and to finally satisfy your own unmet childhood needs? Was perhaps the little girl in you, one of your Russian dolls, running the projector for this emotional film? I imagine that this is a perfectly normal and healthy desire, but it is yet one more loss we have to metabolise – that we will never get the chance to potentially right the wrongs of our own upbringing by doing things differently with *our* children.

The Perfect Mother Fantasy

Each of us has a different idea of what kind of 'perfect mother' we were going to be: mine was a sort of skinny rock-chick in faded Levi jeans and a white T-shirt with long hair flowing down her lean back, no make-up, a light tan with a smattering of freckles and a cute baby on her hip. This fantasy takes place in a huge country-meets-city kitchen full of wonderful smells, intelligent talk radio in the background, the book I've just published in view and a cute mop-headed four-year-old at the kitchen table making naive yet insightful remarks.

This fantasy persisted despite the fact that I'm not naturally skinny and haven't been so for a decade now and that far from looking elegant without make-up I probably would have been looking shattered from lack of sleep (I'm a poor sleeper as it is!). Let alone the inconvenient fact that it was hard enough to write this book *without* children! And in reality, a four-year-old with a new sibling would be more likely to be singing nursery rhymes over and over whilst looking for ways to poke a stick in the new baby's eye when my back was turned! But reality? I had no use for it.

The Perfect Children Fantasy

I'm not sure about you, but my shadow life rarely featured a stroppy teenager, a kid on drugs, a two-year-old having a tantrum or a child with learning difficulties or other challenges. It was always some version of *The Partridge Family* or *The Waltons*, but with a British twist.

I could see how 'my' baby would fit into 'my' dream, but in truth that baby was an extension of my dreams of motherhood. In my perfect children fantasy I'd get on brilliantly with my kids because we'd have similar personalities, aspirations and talents – although they'd be good at maths, which I'm not.

This is about as realistic as Disney. But bringing my shadow family into the light meant looking at the reality of being a mother married to an irresponsible artist and chaotic alcoholic whilst trying to run a business, hold a marriage together and bring up children. A lot more like reality TV in fact. My dreams were just that, dreams, and my child would have had their own dreams, which no doubt would have been completely different. If I'd had children, my daughter might have turned out to be a TV-obsessed princess fascinated by make-up and status, whilst my son could have been a non-academic football-mad boy who just wanted to play sport and violent video games. That tomboy daughter with a love of nature, books and the unseen world? A mini me. That creative, delicate and brilliant son? A mini version of my then husband. In truth, I was playing dollies in my mind; it was fun but it came at a high cost to the life I was actually living.

Demolishing the Playhouse

You may never have doubted for a moment that you wanted to become a mother. You may have played with dolls as a child, had names for your children picked out before you were ten years old and known that being a mother was part of your destiny for as long as you can remember. Or you may not have. I didn't.

Looking back on my own childhood games in the playhouse, it was never about being a mother. It was about independence and being in charge.

I know that I made a decision when I was very young that when I grew up I was *never* going to get married and have children. But this wasn't a decision, nor even a free choice really; rather it was a reaction to my own mother's unhappiness. It was also, at a deeper level, somewhere to 'put' my own unhappiness and confusion as a child. Although I couldn't have told you this until my forties, the reason I didn't think I wanted children until I was almost thirty was because I was terrified that having a child meant revisiting the darker moments of my childhood. Subconsciously, I feared that having been brought up by a mother who was still struggling with the wounds of her *own* childhood, I wouldn't really be up to the job.

Ambivalence About Motherhood

Ambivalence about becoming a mother is quite natural. After all, it's a huge risk, a gamble and a lifelong one at that. We need to remember that it's only been just over fifty years since the Pill became widely available,[110] putting contraception into the hands of women. Making a conscious decision to stop contraception and try to get pregnant is not something that women have yet had much psychological experience with – and it's a decision that we can't entirely rely on logic and common sense to make. We want to be sure that it's a good idea, but there are no assurances it will be. All we can be certain of is that whatever the outcome, there's no turning back. Almost all other big life decisions, including with whom to form a lifelong partnership, can be revised. But if motherhood turns out not to be right for you, tough. You can give your child up for adoption, but that doesn't mean that you're no longer a mother; you're a mother who gave up her child, and that's another taboo, carrying the label of being a 'bad mother'.

> When I had to come to terms with my partner not wanting to have a child with me, and that therefore I'm definitely not going to be a mother, I felt desperate. I was also really angry. But it was not the fact that I will never be a mother, but rather the suffocating thought that I couldn't change my mind anymore. That option is gone; that road's a dead end. As someone hugely ambivalent

*regarding motherhood and having children in the first place, this
felt incredibly scary. The 'what ifs', the 'I could if I wanted to' were
rendered obsolete. Coming to terms with my own ambivalence was
probably the hardest part in that. Because ambivalence is often
seen as a character flaw, and that was, initially, how I saw it, too.*

Ada: 38, Living with Partner, Germany/USA

There are some women who are so certain from a very young age
that they will *never* want children that they seek medical sterilisation in
their twenties, but they often have a very hard time finding a surgeon
who will agree to do so. The idea that they are bound to change their
minds one day is so entrenched in our culture that doctors don't want
to take the risk of depriving them of children at a later date. It seems
that our pronatalist culture literally can't conceive of a woman who is
absolutely sure that she doesn't want children – considering her to be,
in some profound way, 'unnatural'.

The ideology of pronatalism is so strong in many cultures that
we are led to believe that it is 'natural' for *all* women to want to have
children, and that there is something wrong with them if they don't.
Yet if this were a scientific fact, the instinct to have a child would be
something intrinsically biological (like hunger or thirst) and would
exist for every single human female. And it simply doesn't. In fact, the
whole concept of both the 'maternal instinct' and the 'biological clock'
have very little or no basis in science, but are much more sociological
constructs. In *Selfish, Shallow and Self-Absorbed: Sixteen Writers on the
Decision NOT to have Kids*, published in 2015, Laura Kipnis says:

> The 'maternal instinct' is, for example: ... an invented concept
> that arises in a particular point in [Western] history – circa the
> Industrial Revolution, just as the new industrial-era sexual division
> of labour was being negotiated, the one where men go to work and
> women stay at home.[111]

The biological clock wasn't heard of before the twentieth century and
the arrival of freely available contraception and women's emancipation

from almost automatic childbearing. It's a brilliant image because it fits with our time-poor culture and suggests that the closer we get to the bottom of our egg store, the louder such a clock would 'tick'. But it doesn't exist in biology and it would be more accurate to describe it as pronatalism's 'social clock'. And perhaps the very fact that we can think about *not* having a baby proves that it's not an instinct. After all, we can't choose *not* to be hungry or thirsty by thinking differently ...

I'm not trying to downplay how real the concept of the biological clock can feel when you're in a period of babymania, but it does seem that we are 'putting biological language to what is psychological', as the 1970s, researcher and psychoanalyst Dr Frederick Wyatt said.[112] I don't know about you, but it would have been a great support to me during those last few 'still hopeful' years had I known that I was dancing to pronatalism's beat rather than being totally tuned into my own. And as for the idea that not wanting to be a mother is in some way psychologically unhealthy, as Laura Carroll writes in her fascinating book, *The Baby Matrix*:

> Pronatalism has told us that having children is a sign of psycho-logical health. However, the truth is that having children doesn't automatically mean we have our psychological selves together. If that were true, we'd see more troubled non-parents than parents in counseling rooms and prison cells.[113]

As a childless woman, I sometimes answer the 'Why don't you have kids?' question with, 'I couldn't,' which, although it's only part of the story, is usually enough information. But if your answer is, 'I didn't want them,' it's frequently a whole different conversation, mainly because the prejudices that some people have about childless women (but which they don't say to our face) are often freely spoken to the childfree. Statements such as, 'But you won't know what it is to be a woman until you've given birth,' or 'Isn't that rather selfish?' or 'Who's going to look after you when you're old? You'll regret it then!'

The pronatalist belief that it is every woman's destiny to become a mother plays out differently in the lives of childfree and childless women. However, surely it is much better that women who are *absolutely sure* they don't want children can honour that self-awareness rather than end up as reluctant mothers, which is rarely a good outcome for anyone involved? Perhaps our culture's abhorrence of their 'unnaturalness' or 'selfishness' says more about many people's fear of not fitting in to the status quo than it does about childfree adults' own self-awareness and self-definition ...

The Non-Decision That Becomes a Decision

Unrecognised ambivalence, which often 'hides' in the deferral of a decision about motherhood until it's a non-decision which becomes a decision, appears to be a common experience for women who find themselves childless in their forties and can't quite work out how it happened. Having convinced themselves that a baby was something that was 'just going to happen' or that 'the right person was going to come along', or that they'd 'conceive when the time was right', they remained in denial about the approaching end of their fertility.

However, if they tried to express their 3 a.m. thoughts (or 'the hour of the wolf' as James Hollis calls it[14]) most often all they'd hear back from others would be echoes of, 'Don't worry, the right person will come along', 'Just relax', or some other version of a fairy-tale ending.

Some women move into their thirties confident that this is the decade they'll become mothers but, due to circumstances mostly outside their control (jobs, relationships, health, money, housing, fertility, economy, parental illness, etc.), it doesn't happen, and still doesn't happen. As they are, at some deep level, fundamentally unclear about whether they really want a baby or not, they let 'the universe' decide for them. But the universe mirrors back to them their own ambivalence, and so it remains unclear. (Deferring to the universe is the latest get-out-of-jail-free card for really sticky decisions.) Then as their forties loom on the horizon they may realise that they're running out of time and might start making frantic efforts to have a baby before it's too late, getting so caught up in the panic that they *still* don't take the time to get to the bottom of their ambivalence. Babymania takes over from ambivalence and the roots of those feelings remain unexplored. The panicky mantra seems to be, 'What if I really *do* want a child and I don't find out until it's too late?' which once again reasserts the pronatalist idea that if you want a baby and you don't get one, you'll never be able to recover from it.

For some, this mad dash ends with a baby. For others it doesn't. But the ambivalence over becoming a mother goes underground as a taboo once you've had a child. Mothers, you see, aren't 'allowed' to wonder if having children was a good idea, although many of them do. In a National Parenting Survey in the USA, conducted by Oprah's Dr Phil in 2003 with over 20,000 respondents, 40 per cent of parents said that if they knew then what they know now, they wouldn't make the same choice,[115] and according to Laura Carroll, 'anonymous surveys of parents have shown even higher percentages'.[116] In 2013, an article in Britain's *Daily Mail* newspaper went viral after a mother of fifty-seven wrote that her son was 'five days old when the realisation hit me like a physical blow: having a child had been the biggest mistake of my life'.[117] Articles are still being written about that piece, and parents regularly 'confess' similar feelings on anonymous 'confession' websites.[118]

One of my childfree-by-choice friends tells me that when, upon request, she explains her decision to mothers they frequently 'confess' (their word) that, if they had their time again, they wouldn't have had their children. Much as they love them, they've come to realise that motherhood's not what they thought it would be, that they've lost their identity and that they've become 'invisible'. Perhaps it's a social taboo to say that to anyone who's childless because either it makes them sound like they don't love their children, or perhaps it would seem insensitive to say it to us in particular. Because life isn't that simple: mothers can love their children and still dislike taking on the grinding, relentless domestic tasks of motherhood (see Rebecca Asher's *Shattered*[119] for an insider's view), but that human, nuanced complexity seems to get lost in the pronatalist propaganda. Some mothers know it, and may share this 'dark secret' with other mothers – it seems they're just not allowed to speak of it with anyone else. Their current social script reads, 'It's the most fulfilling thing I've ever done,' just as ours reads, 'I'll never get over not being a mother.' But neither of these black-and-white statements are true.

For those last-dashers who *don't* end up with a baby, unexplored ambivalence can become yet another stick with which to beat themselves up. Perhaps they tell themselves that it didn't happen because they didn't *really* want a baby. This is a kind of magical thinking – thinking that if we'd wanted a baby 'harder' it would have worked out differently, taking the idea of positive thinking to an irrational conclusion. Perhaps they think that if they'd been clearer in their desires when they were younger they would have made different decisions, and there's some possible truth in that, but it's a bitter and pointless one because you can't go back and do it differently. I also know plenty of women who've been very, very sure from an early age of their desire to become mothers, and it hasn't worked out for them either. How can you tell a woman who's endured multiple rounds of IVF that she obviously didn't *really* want children or it would have happened? The fact is, there are no guarantees that we get what we want or think we deserve in life. Despite the kind of thinking promoted by books like *The Secret* and which the fertility industry has latched onto, we are not nearly as in control of our lives as it would be comforting to believe.

The Gifts of Ambivalence

There's nothing wrong with us if we were ambivalent about having children. I'll repeat that, because it's so important:

There's nothing wrong with us if we were ambivalent about having children.

Ambivalence shows that, at some deep level, we were truly considering the reality of parenting and whether or not it was the kind of lifelong commitment we could really cope with or be good at. We were thinking of our children's lives as well as our own. Ambivalence about having children is intelligence and compassion in action. It does not mean we were not fit to be mothers, no matter *what* you've convinced yourself of, and however it affected the decisions and non-decisions that contributed to your childlessness.

> *I think wanting to be a mother is not an either/or question. Sure, there are some or many who have always wanted children (though how many stopped to wonder why they always wanted them and where that desire came from?). There are others who have always been clear that they don't want kids. I also suspect that many women (possibly me too) were somewhere in the middle: ambiguous, unsure, wanting them and not wanting them at different points along the way. Sometimes I feel like a fish out of water ... I am neither clearly straightforwardly childfree or clearly straightforwardly childless, but I do suspect this is not uncommon ... at this point whatever I was or am is not so important anymore because I am happy to be where I am and it doesn't really matter whether it's 'less' or 'free'.*
>
> Eimear: 44, Single, Ireland

Within your ambivalence may be the seeds of your recovery from an unhappily childless life. Having those thoughts meant that you were, to some degree, conscious that there were possibilities for you in life *other* than becoming a mother. Having those thoughts may have felt disloyal to your dream, but now that you're looking to get your Plan B going, they may well blossom into a meaningful and fulfilling life without children.

If we begin to explore our ambivalence for the options that we worried about giving up, we will begin to find its gifts. It's time to stop feeling guilty about our ambivalence and instead celebrate our ability to dream alternative dreams.

For millennia there have been women who have had dreams other than that of motherhood and it has been impossible for them to fulfil them. That's not the case anymore. Once we put down the unholy trinity of guilt, shame and blame, we too can start to live out other dreams of how to be a woman in this world.

Decluttering Your Dreams

This is a ritual that is best done with another childless woman or a group. However, it's also very powerful done alone or with your partner, if they are willing.

- Get some really lovely, precious writing paper, an envelope and a pen you really enjoy writing with.
- Write a letter to the child or children you longed to have. This is a goodbye letter to them. In it, you can say whatever you wish in order to feel that you have said your goodbye.
- If you had names picked out for him or her, address them by name in the letter.
- When you have finished your letter, put it in the envelope, seal it and write their names, or whatever you wish, on the outside.
- When the time is right – it may not be straightaway – go to a place outdoors that is special or sacred to you in some way. It might be your own garden; it could be a beach you have memories of, a park ... all that matters is that is feels right to you.
- Take with you your sealed envelope, a tea candle and matches and a tin or plastic container, along with some tissues.
- Either alone, with another childless woman, or with a group standing in a circle, open and read out your letter.

- Once everyone who is present has either read or not read their letter out loud (some might prefer not to), one by one go to the centre of the circle, light your candle, and set fire to your letter. Make sure it's well alight and leave it in the centre of the circle.

- In silence, together, witness the letters burning until they are nearly gone.

- If it feels appropriate, say some blessings and goodbyes to the children in the letters. I usually ask each woman present to say out loud 'Goodbye [name]' and then the whole group says 'Goodbye [name]', which has proved to be very powerful.

- When the ashes have cooled a little, scoop up a portion in your container and take them home with you. You may wish to scatter them, keep them, throw them into flowing water or plant them under a tree dedicated to your children. You may wish to take some photographs of the ashes before you do so.

- Please leave your ritual location as you found it, rubbing away any ashes or marks of fire. If it's a place where having an open fire would be frowned upon or not permitted, consider taking a metal container like a bowl or barbeque tray to contain the fire and leave no marks.

After this ritual, it's good to have something planned with other childless women, if possible, or with your partner if you have one, and if they are willing to be involved. Going out together for something to eat or drink feels like a very ancient way for the living to honour those no longer present. For those of us who don't have anyone to mourn with, this can bring up extra grief, so please make sure to have someone to talk with about how the ritual has affected you – perhaps online as part of a community of childless women or maybe with a therapist.

Even if this feels like a silly idea, please honour your dream of motherhood by letting it go with love and ritual. Our culture has become devoid of rituals, apart from those for marriage, parenting and death, but it's a deep human need and we are a poorer culture for having lost so many of them. As childless women we are each painfully aware that we miss out on the milestones and rituals of family life so our need for this one is even greater. By creating this opportunity to let go, you are honouring yourself and the family you once dreamed of having.

If you have any keepsakes or baby clothes or anything that you've been saving for your children, now or soon might be the time to think of passing them on to someone who can use them. If you have a book or folder on your computer with possible baby names, it's time to let those go too, along with any information you were keeping about IVF, any leftover drugs or paraphernalia, and anything else that you know was related to your dream of motherhood. Only you will know what to keep and what to let go of at this time, so trust yourself, and if there's something you can't bear to be parted from just yet, keep it, and revisit this exercise in a year's time.

Just as we need to declutter our life, we need to declutter our dreams. Without letting go, there can be no space in our life and heart for a new dream. It's time to let go. Let go with love.

Reflections on Chapter 7

In this chapter we've begun to explore how much we may have lost during our years of living as a shadow mother. This can be incredibly painful. If you find feelings of shame and regret surfacing, be very gentle with yourself and trust that you did the best you could at the time. If you are really giving yourself a hard time about this, you might want to jump ahead to Chapter 9 and begin to acquaint yourself with the concept and tools of 'self-compassion'.

We've also looked at some of the fantasies we've been holding onto about the family we longed to have and how perfect we imagined it would have been. Although we may see *now* how absurd some of this was, it's important not to beat yourself up about it – after all, they're called 'fantasies' for a reason . . .

We then began exploring how our own childhood may have influenced our decisions about motherhood, and how those ideas may have fed into any ambivalence we felt about becoming mothers in the first place.

Beginning to lift the lid on parts of our life that we may not have thought about for a long time can be painful. As you've probably worked out by now, it's not an excuse to beat yourself up. You're building up a detailed picture of how and why you got to where you are today, not so that you have more ammunition to prove how dumb you've been, but rather to understand things more fully. Because, buried in the dark, hidden in those places that we don't want to look, are also the very things we need to dig out, polish and bring into the light of our new lives. As Carl Jung said, 'The gold is in the dark.'

Exploring how some of our beliefs about motherhood being 'natural' are hugely influenced by the social construct of pronatalism can be both shocking and liberating. I didn't even know the word pronatalism before I left the babymania phase and started exploring childfree thinking and writing. I was shocked to realise how much I'd been conditioned by this ideology, and how miserable it had made me as a result. And yet there was a part of me that didn't want to believe it. Sometimes it's hard to find out that something you've based so much of your thinking on wasn't true ... It took me a while of dipping my toe back into childfree thinking before I felt comfortable with it ...

If you did the 'Decluttering Your Dreams' exercise, I hope you found it a moving and worthwhile experience. When I do this exercise with groups, there are a lot of tears and it has a profound effect on both the individuals and the group. Be very gentle with yourself in the week following this ritual, as it seems to have a healing effect that can feel quite disruptive at first, sometimes creating a deep tiredness, vivid dreams and/or sleep disturbances, before leading often to a sense of peace and an 'ending' to a period of our life in preparation for the life to come.

If you weren't yet able, for whatever reason, to do this ritual, please consider doing so at a later date, when you feel ready and perhaps when you've got someone to accompany you. The reason that all human cultures have rituals is that their symbolism makes visible the invisible transitions from one stage of our lives to another. Your dreams of a family may have been such a big part of your life that their passing deserves to be honoured with tenderness and witnessed with respect as you move on to the next stage of your life. As do you.

You don't
HAVE
a body;
YOU
ARE
a body.

———

CHAPTER 8

Reconnecting to Your Source

How Your Recovery from Childlessness Affects Your Relationships with Yourself and Others

Perhaps only other women who have experienced involuntary childlessness can comprehend how completely betrayed by life some of us feel. I sometimes imagine that mothers who tragically lose a child may experience a similar loss, but one so much better understood than ours. I know that some of us even envy the fact that they have someone to mourn, that their grief and loss is culturally recognised and that they know what it is to be a mother. But spare a thought for the fact that they too are expected to 'get over it', as if it were flu, a heartlessness which I could never have imagined, but which many bereaved mothers and therapists have since told me about.

To be childless, when for many years you may have reserved a place in your heart, soul and life for a family, is a loss that's hard for others to comprehend. Sometimes, I wonder what it would have been like to have known since childhood that having children was impossible – as it is for those who are born without a womb or have conditions diagnosed in puberty that mean they will never be fertile. I fantasised that, had that been the case for me, I wouldn't have shaped such a huge chunk of my adult hopes around becoming a mother. But then, as I've got to know women for whom this is their reality, I've heard heartbreaking stories of how challenging it can be to become a woman when you know you will never be able to get pregnant naturally, so wrapped up is womanhood with the identity of motherhood.

At some deep level, part of the devastation of childlessness is that we feel a profound sense of being betrayed by life, by our bodies and by ourselves.

The shift in identity from being a woman who hopes, one day, to become a mother to one who knows, without question, that it's never going to happen is so huge that it throws *everything* into question. This life-changing threshold is invisible to others and, as yet, little understood or spoken about; but those of us living through it know that it's perhaps the toughest challenge we've faced so far.

We may be dealing with a deep sense of betrayal of ourselves by ourselves, and this can lead us to question the very nature of our relationship with ourselves, our bodies and our belief systems. Those who haven't experienced this sometimes accuse me of exaggerating how it feels, but I'm not. These are our truths and sometimes they are extreme. During this process we may also find that every other relationship in our life comes under scrutiny too! This next little exercise will hopefully help to show why that is.

EXERCISE 9
Going Dotty

Grab a piece of paper (you can also do it in your head, but it's very quick and works best on paper).

Imagine all the relationships in your life as a sort of map made up of dots. You are a dot at the centre and around you, also represented by dots, are your key relationships – your partner, family, friends, colleagues, etc. If you draw a line between your dot and each of the other dots, every line will be a different length and at a different angle to 'you'.

Now, imagine that you move the dot representing yourself to a different place – even by the tiniest amount. See what happens to the lines? By moving yourself even the slightest bit, you are at a different angle and distance from absolutely everyone else in your life.

So, along with the internal changes we're dealing with, it may seem like we also have to contend with what can feel like an endless amount of change in *all* our relationships. Because you are not the same person you were when you made the subconscious contracts that form the basis for your current relationships, you may find that your relationships start to feel like they're not quite working anymore. And so, for everyone involved, these contracts will need to be renegotiated. This isn't easy for most of us, because it requires making explicit what may have been implicit before, and probably involves some really frank heart-to-hearts.

This can be incredibly hard on those around us too. Because it may be that what they thought and felt was a secure relationship contract with you is one *you've* now decided has to be renegotiated. Unilateral moves like this can seem pretty unfair to others. After all, from where they're standing they may feel that not only have they supported you through some of the most difficult years of your life, but now that you're coming out the other side, there's a whole new set of problems to be got through! But that's life – always on the move, always changing. When a plant stops growing, it dies and so do people, in more subtle ways.

Fully accepting my partner's decision not to have a child with me has had a big effect on our relationship. When you don't have to focus on securing the source for potential offspring, things naturally change and it depends on you in which direction that change goes. You can be forever angry and miserable, or leave and try to find another partner, or you can simply take the risk of working through it. I find that our relationship has become even more than it was before. It's not about having children together; it is about being together. The focus now rests on the depth and quality of our relationship, which is not merely a by-product of something else; it is the first and only focus.

Ada: 38, Living with Partner, Germany/USA

The process of healing from loss is a process of change. I imagine it as an expansion of our identity until it's big enough to include and integrate that loss. Grieving changes us and we are never the same again after loving someone or grieving someone.

When couples lose a child, the impact of that bereavement can break up the relationship. This is also true for other big life transitions as well, like when one partner becomes sober and deals with the issues that led to them drinking too much. And for couples who are coming to terms with the end of their trying-to-conceive journey or who have suffered miscarriage, early-term loss or stillbirth, or perhaps are trying to move forward without children because one partner has changed their mind about having children, or for any of the many reasons we find ourselves without the child we expected, this loss can become a major stumbling block to continued connection.

In my case, it probably had something to do with the relationship's demise. I wasn't given the chance to renegotiate because in my miscarriage grief, I wasn't aware that my ex had gone off with another.

Claude: 44, Single, UK

Such losses, so huge to process, may become so difficult to talk about that they become a block in the relationship, and perhaps, in the end, it may seem easier to split up than to work out what to do about the baby elephant in the room.

Intimacy and honesty are, in fact, the same thing.

Faced with this, couples may turn away from each other or enter into a 'pretend' intimacy – a sort of intimacy-lite – which doesn't fool either of them for long, but may be thought of perhaps as the denial stage of their grieving process as a couple. For many couples, the necessary anger stage of grief is one that they don't feel able to deal with together; or conversely they may be so angry that they destroy the relationship by taking it out on each other. In order to do our grief work *within* our primary relationship we will need support from *outside* that relationship.

As well as our relationship with our partner (if we have one), our relationships with family, friends and colleagues may also go through a change. Now that you've officially either given up trying or have made some kind of public declaration that you've accepted that it's not going to happen for you, people may well breathe a big sigh of relief and expect things to 'get back to normal'. But there is no 'normal' to go back to. I spent fifteen years of my life longing to be a mother, realising at forty-four and a half that it was not to be and falling headfirst into my grieving process. But even the fact that I'd given up didn't stop people continuing to bombard me with miracle baby stories, and they still do. These days it's more often the 'Why don't you just adopt?' comment (don't you just love that 'just'!) rather than the 'Don't give up, you never know, it's never too late', but they're not based in any reality. It doesn't seem to occur to them that as a single, self-employed person I have neither the time nor the financial or logistical resources to adopt. And anyway, as someone who has written publicly about her grief and depression over childlessness I would not be considered a suitable candidate – just imagine how it would be for an adopted child to read all that one day ... I do know childless single women and couples who've adopted, but I've also lost count of the number of financially and emotionally stable couples I know of who've been turned down as adoptive parents, or who've been approved, but after years of waiting for a match have given up. Indeed, Gateway Women runs a private online support community solely for members going through the adoption process.[120] There's only so much hope and heartbreak you can live with before you realise that your sanity is hanging on by a thread. As Lisa Manterfield writes about her and her husband's decision not to pursue adoption, 'We maxed out the heartbreak cards already.'[121]

The reality is that surviving and thriving after childlessness changes every aspect of our life and relationships. Colleagues who may have leaned on us when they were overstretched may find that we're not so willing to put in the overtime any more. Siblings who've expected us to be their always available babysitter may be confused when we develop other priorities. Friends may find our new energy and commitment to things that they're not interested in (or don't have the time for as parents) confronting and difficult. And our partners may not know who we are anymore. And we're not sure yet, either.

Coming to terms with our childlessness as a permanent identity is a shift that changes everything and everyone around us. It's important to recognise that and to be understanding of other people's reactions and to make allowances for them, if possible. Some of our relationships may dissolve as we grow and change and find new relationships that suit us better. Some relationships will evolve along with us.

The fact is, not everyone *wants* to be as potentially free of illusion and as emotionally and psychologically mature as we are having to become. And it's neither our right nor our job to tell them that they must. There's also no need to jettison relationships that don't seem to be working anymore as part of the emotional house clearance you may be embarking upon. It may well be that although we're moving away from those people at the moment, we are travelling in a very big spiral with our healing and it's a relationship we might be able to reconnect with again one day.

Some Tips for Relationship Renegotiation

- Be gentle with yourself and others throughout this process of relationship renegotiation.

- Learning to actively practise self-compassion will help you, and others, deal with the changes (more on that in Chapter 9).

- Be honest about what you're going through and ask for patience and tolerance from others, and give it back twice over. Childlessness is a taboo and others may be scared and uncomfortable around us; educate them in how to support you rather than expecting them to be mind-readers.

- Stop expecting others to understand your situation. In answer to a question I put to Brené Brown at a public talk in July 2013,[122] infertility and childlessness has shown up in her research as 'the number one area of empathy failure'. Your friends and family are not *uniquely* unable to understand!

- Recognise that you don't yet know who you're becoming – you're a work in progress. Try not to make any irrevocable decisions for a couple of years at least. Grieving changes us in surprising (and often wonderful) ways.

- Understand that your grieving and healing affects everyone and everything around you. Even if you're *not* talking about it, it has a shape and presence that can be challenging for others to cope with as it may bring *their* ungrieved losses to the surface.

- Accept that no one else will change to your timetable. No one. Even if they promise they will. Focus on your own healing.

- It's OK to 'park' a friendship or relationship if it's too hot to deal with right now – you don't need to be an emotional ninja. Sometimes a 'cooling off' period works for everyone and once you feel a bit clearer about things you (and they) can take it from there.

- Get support from outside your primary relationships and give the people in your intimate circle a rest from your issues. This is when the sisterhood of other childless women can be so powerful.

Time to Stop Punishing Yourself

Living with a body that we felt was 'meant' to have children can be hard once that dream is over. Sometimes it's easier to disconnect from it altogether. We may have put our bodies through hellish medical procedures, only to end up with empty bank accounts, broken bodies and broken dreams. We may have made ourselves sick with hope, that most toxic of fertility drugs. We may have endured miscarriages, early-term loss or stillbirth, or we may never have got pregnant. We may have nurtured our bodies through decades of menstruation – been disciplined and honourable with our birth control, taken vitamins, kept fit, eaten a healthy diet and treated ourselves as mothers-to-be – only to never even have had the *chance* to try for a baby. I have become aware from the women I have worked with that those who have never had this chance can feel at the 'bottom of the pile' of childless-by-circumstance women, judging themselves on some invisible pecking order of shame and denying themselves even the right to feel *included* in the collective pain of childless women.

And these days, now that we know we will never be mothers, we may be ignoring our body altogether to the point of neglect.

Body? What body? I felt cut off from my body for several years. It was as though I was just a head, somehow moving around the world on an independent vehicle underneath.

Marjon: 43, Engaged, The Netherlands

What's the point of these breasts if they will never feed a child? This rounded belly if it will never keep a growing baby safe? These hips if they were never meant for childbirth? What's the point of having a womanly body at all?

We may be peri-menopausal or into the menopause, our skin, hair and hormones reminding us that our girlish days are well and truly behind us. The periods that tied us to the rhythm of the moon, like the mysterious creatures we are, now quieting, or flooding, or silent. I have written of the experience of menopause for childless women as 'a death we survive'.[123] For those of us who have managed (perhaps even unconsciously) to keep some flicker of hope going, the menopause can come as a shocking dose of reality and tip us into profound grief. For some women the menopause comes very early, in their teens, twenties or thirties, and brutally cuts short their dreams of motherhood. And then there are those childless women who experience immediate surgical menopause after total hysterectomies for whom the force of the grief can be overwhelming and, sadly it seems, rarely treated with empathy by medical professionals.

> *As I was only thirty-two when my menopause began, I was very much alone on this path. Doctors laughed at me when I suggested early menopause, refusing to test my hormones until I was thirty-seven. Growing up, everyone talks about puberty for years before you experience it, but no one ever talks about menopause, other than hot flushes and mood swings – it's so cloaked in secrecy and shame. When I needed to have a hysterectomy I wasn't offered counselling, wasn't told what to expect, and wasn't given a follow-up appointment. And afterwards not a single one of my friends called or came to visit; they were all too busy with their families.*
> Jenni: 40, Single, Australia

We may be living in our heads these days – staying late at work when we don't really need to, numbing out by watching too much TV, mindlessly checking Facebook and wandering around our homes as if we're looking for something that we left somewhere, but just can't quite remember what it is, or where we put it. We have lost our connection to source.

Our body is our spirit made flesh. Whatever your faith or whether you have no faith, if you wanted to have a child you know that there is something sacred about a woman's body and its ability to bring forth life and you feel denied *your* part in that sacrament.

But you were a sacred birth once. You are still sacred.

By blaming our body we internalise the shame and rage we feel about how things have worked out for us; we bury it alive in our flesh. We wall ourselves in with it. It is easier to grab the flesh on our hips and say, 'I'm disgusting,' than it is to feel the grief contained in our lost hopes for those curves, that womanly fat.

It is easier to stop caring about our body, eat rubbish food and never take any exercise than it is to work through our sense of having failed and being unable to imagine a future that fills us with any sense of hope or excitement.

It's easier to deny ourselves bodily pleasure, to withdraw from the body, to withdraw from sex with our partner or find it hard to enjoy it as we once did, to give up looking for a relationship and resign ourselves to celibacy, to starve and over-exercise as a way of punishing ourselves, than it is to feel the pain of our crushing betrayal by life.

Our body is sacred, but *we* don't feel worthy of that sacrament anymore.

Forgiving Your Body

Forgiving our body is forgiving ourselves for 'getting it wrong', for 'failing', for every 'stupid decision' we made that got us to the place we are today. For the illnesses and inheritances that made it too difficult or impossible to have a baby. For the wanderings and wonderings of our early womanhood while we tried to work out who we were, before we could even think about becoming mothers.

We need our bodies to have that future – we're not going to get there by thought alone! But we can't dump so much of the pain from our unmet longings into our flesh and then expect it to spring into action, reborn, revitalised and ready to go once we're ready to move towards our Plan B. Our body is not a tool, there to carry out our wishes; it *is* our wishes. Every thought, every dream, every experience is written on our body, in our body.

Forgiving our body is an act of grace that frees us up to start imagining that we have a future again. That we <u>deserve</u> a future again.

It has been said that, 'We are not human beings having a spiritual experience; we are spiritual beings having a human experience.'[124]

The fact is, however you look at it, the 'you' that is reading this book is bigger than this body, these mistakes, these unlucky breaks, this heartbreak. And thus you can transcend and transform this pain into a new and passionate life. This is the gift of being both spirit and body, yoked by a creative mind.

But first, you have to forgive your body. Deep down, we know that there's healing to be done. And we fear that healing as much as we long for it. In Chapter 4 we started exploring our grief around our childlessness and letting that process of healing move through us. Now we also need to mourn our youth, our strength, our fertility. There is more to us than these bodies, but we can't do anything without them. However much you want to deny that you have a body, it's not going to go away whilst you live. As long as you deny your body the love it craves, you are denying yourself the support you need to move forward. You can't drag your body with you, reluctantly. You've got to make this trip together, willingly.

Allowing yourself to grieve the losses your body has lived through with you will allow it to heal, and as *it* heals, *you* heal. As you change, your body changes with you. Because your body *is* you.

Because you don't have a body; you <u>are</u> a body.

Learning to Love Your Body Again

Right now, you may be wondering what the hell I'm on about – *has she gone all beardy-weirdy on me now?* But this idea that our bodies *are* us, not some machine that we control, strikes at the very heart of the mind–body duality that has dominated Western thinking since the Enlightenment. Science is beginning, with its explorations into quantum realms, to accept the idea that there is an intelligence at work in our bodies and in the universe which is non-rational and immensely smart. And perhaps even non-local in some instances too.

We are not dumb flesh run by a smart computer. We are spirit (intelligence if you prefer) made flesh – and way cleverer than the smartest computer. Forgiving our body is not mere lip service to some new-age idea. It has immense power.

> *For many years I had strong negative feelings towards my body as I blamed it for not being good enough to attract a man and failing me in not having a child. Now I am ageing I am a lot more tender and caring towards it. I realise what a miracle it is that I have lived in this precious body for over fifty years and it has hardly failed me. I try to take good care of it these days and not beat myself up on those days that I don't.*
>
> Natasha: 50, Single, UK

Loving your body is an act of profound acceptance and healing that will strengthen and support you as you learn to cherish yourself and your life again. I'm not suggesting the kind of regime that you might find in a women's magazine, but rather a conscious decision to offer gratitude to your body for getting you this far and a willingness to be grateful to it in the future. If this body had borne children, flesh of your flesh, how tenderly would you regard the flesh of your children?

It's time to stop denying yourself the love you deserve. It is the same flesh that your children would have been made of.

The body that you love and feel at home in already exists. You don't have to create it by your own will. It is there, you just have to remember it and then find your way back to it.

There is a place in your memory, I hope, of a time when you were a young girl, before you divorced yourself from your body, when you and your flesh moved and thought and felt as one. For me, it is a memory of standing ankle-high in a babbling brook with a butterfly net in my hand, fishing for the tiny sticklebacks darting around the rocks. The sun is on my back and dancing on the water, while the shadow of the footbridge lies dark and cool behind me. I am totally absorbed in the bright, laughing water and my body moves with me like a silent wriggling fish. We are one.

This union is our birthright, yet our culture, wonderful in so many ways, has also created a glory in the artificial, the easy to spot, the flashy. But these moments of poise and stillness when our spirit and body breathe together and know each other to be true, this honest joining is the kind of bodily integrity on which new dreams can be built.

Finding Your Source

Each of us, regardless of our beliefs, lack of beliefs, our religious views and observances or not, *has* to find a way back to source.

What Is Source?
Source is the endless boundlessness of our spirit, our intelligence, our essential self. Some think of it as 'spirit', but 'life force' or 'universal intelligence' may sit better with you. Now before you back off from the page, I'm not asking you to believe anything 'woo woo'. But I would like to invite you to believe that you are more than your childlessness.

And to do that, you need to stop, be quiet and listen to your body and to the sweet simplicity of your nature under all your negative beliefs and broken dreams.

There is a space at the core of us all, a deep pool of quietness filled with love. It took me a long time to connect with it after the knocks and dramas of life, but when I found my way back there, I realised that I was home again. Moreover, after a while, I came to understand that where I go is not a *place* at all. I am already there. It *is* me, and I am it. Connecting with it gives me a boundless sense of freedom, curiosity, joy and compassion and when I was a child I knew it as intimately as the scene from my bedroom window.

The contemplative part of all religions and philosophies comes from source. Most of us in Western culture become gradually disconnected from it at some point, and although many of us may continue to have faith of some kind and perhaps may even be observant of that faith, few of us remain in daily contact with the source of that faith.

> *I'm Christian, an Episcopalian, and during the brunt of my grief I was really doing the 'fake it till you make it' kind of thing, but I still went to church and was very open with our priest about how pissed off I was that God left us childless while my drug-addicted cousin gave birth to her second child at forty. My prayer life is much deeper now, but it's different. I used to do all the talking before, now I just listen for God's voice . . . and He is there.*
>
> Kyla: 43, Married, USA

You don't have to believe in anything to have access to source; it runs through everything and everyone and is our birthright. We are all made of the same material that fires the sun and unfurls the buds of spring. We are all made of source; we are all part of source.

Creativity comes from source; love comes from source; compassion comes from source; forgiveness comes from source; hope and resilience come from source. We come from source. We are source.

We are *massively* going against the grain of our culture by daring to give birth to ourselves anew as a way to recover from our childlessness. It is an act of colossal courage and given little regard, respect or credence by most others. There is very little support, hardly any recognition and no award ceremonies for remaking our lives around a new core of meaning. As I've said before, culturally no one really cares much what we do with our lives now as long as we pay our taxes, keep quiet and take care of sick and elderly relatives. Because of this, we need to gather our support for the changes we're going through from a deeper place and from each other.

Buddhism has made me very aware that I'm part of a larger whole. Nowadays, I prefer to seek out my own way of reconnecting. Nature is a good one for me. Animals too. I'm part of a huge living organism that doesn't die when I die. I read somewhere that human consciousness is a way for the universe to witness itself. I like that. Just being a witness and enjoying the beauty of this world is very healing. And a good antidote for the existential pain that comes with childlessness.

Marjon: 43, Engaged, The Netherlands

Even our partners, family and closest friends may disagree or ridicule what we're trying to do. The fact is, when someone, anyone, chooses to consciously heal, this can be very challenging for those around them. Because as we heal, it touches the desire in *them* to heal and, rather than it inspiring them, they may feel guilty about their own resistance and project that back onto us as hostility, cynicism and ridicule.

So, expect some flak from others as you begin to change. In fact, you might find that it's better to keep quiet about what you're up to in the early stages, when it's so easy to be knocked off course by an unsupportive or critical remark from someone we care about. Instead, seek the support of people interested and active on a path of personal transformation and if they're also childless women, all the better!

The support of other childless women and a connection to source are, in my experience, vital to get your healing project on the road. In time, others will want what you've got, but until you've got it, they're unlikely to give you any help or support to get it. No one believes a prophet in their own land. Keep quiet and let others notice how 'well you're looking these days', how much 'happier' or 'calmer' you seem.

You don't need to convert anyone, or convince anyone. Just do your thing, and shine.

Each of us connects to source in our own way and it might take a bit of experimentation to find the way that works for you and is sustainable. It's all very well going away on a meditation retreat and feeling all pure and 'spiritual' on the journey home, but if you can't fit it around your day-to-day life, it's not a reliable way for you to connect to source.

If we are to open ourselves up to the possibility of a meaningful and fulfilling life without children, we need to connect to source in a way that works for us, as often as we can. I recommend daily.

Opening Up Your Connection to Source

Here are some suggestions taken from my own experience of reading, experimenting, failing, starting again, giving up, losing heart and somehow managing to keep on going. There's more information in the 'Recommended Reading' section of the Appendix if you want to explore further.

- Give up reading women's magazines and watching TV programmes that promote the idea that your body is something to be perfected. Unplug from anything that makes you feel 'less than' (and that includes a lot of social media too). Consume media intelligently and compassionately − would you have let your children get their values this way? Thought not.

- Try Julia Cameron's 'Morning Pages' exercise from her book, *The Artist's Way*.[125]

- Attend twelve-step meetings of any kind. The most well known is Alcoholics Anonymous, but there are meetings for all kinds of issues, including OA (Overeaters Anonymous) for all types of problems with food and DA (Debtors Anonymous), which is for anyone with a cranky relationship with money (not just debt) and, as money and self-worth are closely aligned, it can be really enlightening . . .

- Create something: writing, blogging, painting, gardening, engine-building, home-making, singing, baking, sewing, dancing, poetry . . .

- Take a walk alone in nature (woods and hills do it for me, but for you it might be the beach, or arid plains . . .)

- Try meditating. There are great phone apps to help you get into the habit. Or you might consider an online or in-person mindfulness course.

- Practise self-compassion. Kristin Neff's book *Self-Compassion*[126] is an excellent guide to understanding the power of this approach and why it's very different from selfishness or self-obsession. (You can read more about self-compassion in Chapter 9.)

- Give up perfectionism and embrace your mistakes, failure, bloopers and getting it wrong as part of being human. Brené Brown's my heroine on this one − read *The Gifts of Imperfection*[127] to understand why.

- Find a way to touch the sublime: great architecture, sacred buildings, inspiring art, a magnificent landscape, an astonishing film, moving poetry ... Anything that touches your soul and fills you with a sense of awe, of expansiveness.

- Take some exercise you enjoy (rather than endure). For me the best are yoga, walking, swimming and cycling. But for you it might be football, skydiving, running ...

- Listen to pure birdsong recordings – those without music in the background. I prefer British and European sounds; you might find that a recording from the environment you grew up in has a special quality for you too.

- Speak up in the face of abuse, unkindness or injustice. For me there's nothing like giving my inner warrior an outlet to connect me to a place of power and truth.

- Commit random acts of kindness. Mike Dickson's inspiring book, *Please Take One*,[128] on the power of generosity, is great for ideas.

- Live from a place of integrity, especially when no one is looking.

- Seek out inspirational and spiritual literature from different faiths and traditions.

- Watch TED.com videos of inspirational talks.

- Spend time with people who inspire you, make you laugh, remind you of the best of you and who support you on the path towards your Plan B.

EXERCISE 10
Saying Thank You

Next time you have a shower or bath, take a moment afterwards to show your gratitude to each part of your body as you moisturise it. For many women, even the idea of this exercise repels them – 'But I don't like a single part of my body!' is something I've often heard. The shift to make is that this isn't about *liking* your body; it's about being *grateful* to it. If you find it difficult to access gratitude for a part of your body, think about what your daily life would be like without, for example, your knees, and after that you may find it easier to feel the gratitude ...

The way I do it is that I start with my feet and say thank you to each part of my body in turn in a specific way that's become a bit of ritual for me. It looks a bit crazy when I write it down, but I'll say thank you to my feet 'for supporting me and allowing me to move around my world'; to my knees 'for being so flexible and allowing me to still sit comfortably cross-legged' ... etc. When I get to my bottom, which is larger than I would like, I'll say, 'Thank you for being so comfortable to sit on!'

Perhaps one of the hardest areas for many of us is our stomach area, as not only do we store so much grief here (along with all our emotions), but it can be such a place of sadness around childbearing. At first, feeling gratitude to this part of our body can be particularly hard, so you may wish to focus on your digestive system rather than your reproductive organs to begin with. I usually say, 'Thank you for digesting everything I eat and turning it into nourishment for my life.'

After you've finished this exercise you will hopefully find that your whole body is zinging with energy and that you have a warm glow all over. It's an amazing feeling and the more you do it, the better it gets. The skin is a very sensitive organ and whether it's our own caress or another's, if we stroke our skin tenderly and with full attention it stimulates the flow of oxytocin, the feel-good bonding hormone that we get from a hug or after an orgasm.

If you do this exercise daily, you may begin to feel a softening in any body-hatred or self-shame you might feel, and in turn this may begin to affect what you see when you look in the mirror. I am so much kinder to myself now when I look in the mirror – it's my body and although it doesn't look great in a bikini, I can't say that seems terribly important anymore. My body is my soul's home and, as Geneen Roth would say, 'Your body is the piece of the universe that you've been given to take care of.'[129]

EXERCISE 11

Connecting to Source

Using my suggestions from 'Opening Up Your Connection to Source', do something at least once, and preferably two or three times, in the next week that allows you to connect with the spaciousness of source. If you can do it daily, that would be amazing, but you might need to experiment with several different techniques until you find one that feels right for a daily practice.

The clue is in the word 'spaciousness' – it's the best way I can describe the way my heart and the centre of my chest area 'opens', releasing a sense of freedom and joy. This does not necessarily have to be articulated or classified as a spiritual experience; it's just that I don't know of any widely enough disseminated vocabulary other than 'spiritual' to describe it yet. Martha Beck calls it 'wordlessness' and I like that too.[130]

Reflections on Chapter 8

In this chapter we've been looking at how the process of change brings into focus all our relationships – with our bodies, with our deepest self and with others in our life.

How has it been for you to start thinking about these things? Have you perhaps realised that you've been incredibly hard on yourself up until now and that maybe it's time you cut yourself some slack? Or perhaps you've had some fresh thoughts about how others relate (or fail to relate) to you?

If you managed to do the 'Saying Thank You' exercise, I hope you found it a simple but moving way of beginning to ask your body's forgiveness after years of treating it with disdain or abuse. It may have brought up some strong feelings of sadness or shame, which is to be expected. See if you can do the exercise regularly, and notice how each time you do it, your feelings shift a little ... You might also want to check out some of my additional recommended reading on the subject, particularly the work of Brené Brown (see Appendix).

Sometimes, even the idea of connecting back to source can be very provocative. The depth of betrayal by life that some of us feel might also include a feeling of being betrayed by our beliefs. When bad things happen to good people and we are brought face to face with our powerlessness as human beings, such things can shake us to the core. Whatever your beliefs, a crisis of faith is a profoundly destabilising experience.

Choosing to re-engage with thoughts like this after such a crisis can be very challenging. How was it for you to start exploring these issues, and how do you feel about the idea of reconnecting to source? If you tried the 'Connecting to Source' exercise, how was that? Or did you dismiss it as more ridiculous new-age nonsense? Please remember that source does not have to be explored or experienced in a religious or spiritual context if that's not your thing. Find a way of relating to it that works for you – such as 'life force' or 'universal intelligence', for example – and connect to it in whatever way feels right for you.

Reconnecting to our source is not a one-off experience and you may find, as have I and many other childless women in recovery, that our relationship with source changes as we continue our journey towards and into our Plan B. What works for you may be something in this chapter, or it may not. But there *will* be a way for you to find your way home if you keep looking. If it all feels a bit much right now, perhaps put a date in your diary to come back to this chapter and these exercises in about six months – you may find that something has shifted internally by then and it feels like something you can have another try at.

Self-care
is not
self-indulgence;
self-care is
SELF-RESPECT.

CHAPTER 9

The Mother Within

The Good Mother Archetype

Over the course of our time wanting to be mothers – for some of us from when we were young girls – we have dreamed about mother-hood. We've imagined what kind of mothers we would be, how we would do things differently from (or the same as) our own mothers, what we would name our children, how we would treat them. We see our friends, family and complete strangers parenting their children and think, *I wouldn't do it like that*, or *That's amazing, I'll remember that*. With our nephews, nieces, godchildren and the other children in our life we find ourselves drawing on a deep reservoir of instinct and learned behaviour as we relate to them, nurture them, teach them, comfort them and keep them safe.

There is a part of us that is a mother even though we don't have a child of our own.

In our culture there are often examples of women who are biologic-ally able to give birth but for whom being a parent is psychologically a major challenge. We are their opposite – women who are mothers in spirit, not in reality. We are childless mothers, not just childless women.

In Jungian psychology, an archetype is something that exists as a potential within a personality until activated by the right circumstances, influence or experience. Everyone therefore has a 'mother archetype' and, for those of us who have longed to be mothers, those years of longing may have activated that archetype, yet it has never had a chance to be fully expressed. This may contribute to the 'aching arms' some of us report – a very physically uncomfortable feeling that can be experienced when our desire to nurture has been thwarted. It is something that mothers who lose their children also report experiencing.

This nurturing part of us finds expression in our care towards our loved ones, in mentoring young people, with our pets and with the children in our personal and professional lives.

Ironically, for those of us who work in caring professions and with children, our own wounding has given us a capacity for empathy that is a balm to others. We can be loyal friends, patient daughters, loving partners, sensitive stepmothers, understanding sisters, kind aunts, civilised and friendly exes.

We are good women to others. So why are we so often cruel to ourselves?

Meet Your Inner Bitch

It's a shocking truth that many of us deny ourselves the tenderness and empathy that we so willingly and generously extend towards others. We talk to ourselves and treat ourselves in ways that we would never dream of doing to anyone else.

It seems that for some of us, from the moment we get out of bed there's a toxic running commentary in our head and tuning into it can be a pretty shocking revelation. For a moment, imagine you were to 'turn the speakers on' and start hearing your negative internal commentary out loud . . .

Here are some things that I used to hear in my own head, and some that other women have shared with me:

- You're just not good enough.
- Who put you in charge, you idiot?!
- You look like shit today.
- There's something wrong with you.
- Stupid bitch.
- Loser.
- What's the point of reading this book, of trying to change – you'll never do it.

If you actually, physically, <u>can't</u> say this stuff out loud, you're not alone. Because it may be that you realise that you would <u>never</u> talk like that to anyone. You're just 'not that kind of person'. So what do you think talking to <u>yourself</u> like that is doing to you?!

Some of us don't hear statements like the ones above, but instead 'feel' our Inner Bitch – as if we've been judged somehow and are feeling the physical effect of shame.

It's not just words that I get. I get a sensation of disgust and ridicule without any words being said. The overwhelming message is that there is something wrong with me.

Margot: 67, Married, USA

Wherever your harsh internal voice comes from, and whether you call it your Inner Critic, your Inner Bitch, your Top Dog or just 'you', it's time to understand it a little better in order to form a new and kinder relationship with yourself.

In her book *Self-Compassion*, Kristin Neff explains that the part of the brain that lights up during self-criticism is the amygdala – the oldest part of the human brain and the one that we share with reptiles. It would therefore seem that self-criticism is activated as a response to a perceived threat, as it's triggered by the same part of the brain that makes you jump when you hear a loud noise, even before you've had a chance to work out whether it's anything to worry about or not. Neff goes on to formulate that self-criticism is therefore trying to help and protect us. These days, we don't have to worry much about being eaten by predators, but we do have to 'fit in' and so this primitive 'fight-flight-freeze' response is now used by our modern human brain to deal with social and emotional risks to our status, acceptability and lovability. Unfortunately, it also turns out that as a behaviour modification, self-criticism is, to use the non-scientific term, lousy! Self-kindness, on the other hand, 'allows us to feel safe as we respond to painful experiences, so that we are no longer operating from a place of fear'.[131]

So you see, there's nothing inherently 'wrong' with your Inner Bitch – she has her uses. Her vocabulary and values are created from what you learned from your parents, teachers and primary caregivers. Freud called this part of us our 'superego' and it's a crucial part of what becomes our adult conscience. But it's a building block, not the whole show.

Our Inner Bitch has evolved to keep us safe from harm. But it seems that for many of us she's become a form of self-harm.

John Gottman, an influential American marriage therapist, has shown through hundreds of hours of close video analysis that for every critical comment or piece of feedback a couple gives each other it needs to be balanced with five positive comments or the marriage is in trouble. This 5:1 ratio proved to be accurate in 94 per cent of the marriages Gottman analysed.[132] Interestingly, the same 5:1 ratio has also been shown to be one of the hallmarks of outstanding business teams, with 3:1 being the 'tipping point' between teams failing and beginning to thrive.[133]

Do you give yourself at least five pieces of positive feedback for each critical one? Or even 3:1? Or did a voice pipe up to tell you that if you did that you'd be 'spoiling yourself' or 'going soft', or any of the other messages you may have picked up? We live in a particularly perfectionist- and achievement-oriented culture at the moment, and there's a prevailing idea that 'pushing yourself' is more productive than 'being kind to yourself'. Somewhere along the way, self-compassion has become seen as a form of weakness, when in fact it's a source of incredible inner strength and resilience. Does the Dalai Lama seem like a 'weak' man to you?

> *Self-compassion has not made me soft at all! In fact, while practising self-compassion, I've grown fiercer about protecting my self-interest. I'm not sure all the people around me like that 'new' aspect of me. Self-compassion doesn't make you soft. Self-compassion can make you really tough, ready to set boundaries and protect them. I get angry when people step over my boundaries and I'm not afraid to tell them anymore. Consequently, I can allow myself to be more self-compassionate. It seems like a paradox, but it really makes sense once you pay attention to how it works.*
>
> Marjon: 43, Engaged, The Netherlands

We all know how much a critical comment from someone we love and respect can hurt. So just imagine what criticising *ourselves* harshly and with the relentlessness that many of us have learned *has* done to us and *is* doing to us. It's an act of psychic self-abuse and a way of punishing ourselves for being human and imperfect. Just like everyone else.

For example, when you're tired and need to take a nap, what does your Inner Bitch say? Does she say, 'Sweetheart, you look a bit tired, why don't you take a nap?' or is she more likely to sneer, 'You look like shit, but don't even think about sloping off for a nap – you've got way too much to do. You're just lazy. You shouldn't have stayed up so late last night. It's your own fault. Just get on with it and stop complaining'?

> *My Inner Bitch is in retirement now (almost permanent). The things she used to say to me included 'you stupid cow', 'you are*

pathetic, no wonder you can't have children', 'nothing you do ever lasts, it will just be another fad', 'there's no excuse for being fat, you haven't had a baby', 'what is the point of you?'.

Heather: 40, Married, UK

This kind of relentless internal abuse wears us down, turns us off and puts us into a kind of permanent low-level battle with ourselves. In the end, it may be easier to numb out and try to avoid our inner world altogether than deal with this kind of bullying barrage: turn the TV up louder, have another snack, pour another drink, stay late at work or stay in bed. However, by tuning out our inner world because of our Inner Bitch, we also tune out everything else, and deny ourselves access to joy, creativity, dreams, inspirations, passion and love. This may be a factor contributing to the 'emotional deadness' that so many of us experience and which we fear may be a permanent state for the rest of our lives.

In order to even feel worthy of a meaningful and fulfilling life again, you're going to have to make friends with your Inner Bitch.

I don't know about you, but for me, not having the family I dreamed of somehow confirmed that my Inner Bitch had been right all along; that there was something fundamentally wrong with me that I couldn't even get this simple thing right, something that everyone else seemed to manage, often even by accident! My Inner Bitch wore me into the ground and, fuelled by the dark depression of grief, nearly took me out of the running altogether. There were days when I seriously wondered if I wanted any more of life as it had become so painful, dark and utterly joyless. My inner world, devoid of love, became a torment to me. I hid it well from others, but alone at home I felt I was being eaten alive by my thoughts, my judgements, my criticisms. Each day I would wake up and try to 'get it right', but the bar was always too high and I would 'fail' and feel worthless, often before I'd even finished breakfast, owing to the fact that my food choices weren't 'up to scratch'. It was just toast. Again.

Your Inner Bitch isn't daft or evil; there's often wisdom in your self-criticism too. But there's no wisdom in running yourself down and abusing yourself every moment you're awake. You wouldn't expect a dog to thrive in those circumstances, let alone a human being, let alone a woman recovering from the grief of childlessness and doing her damnedest to build a new life from the wreckage of her dreams.

The thing is, would you have talked to your children like this? (Didn't think so.) But there's a child inside you, and she's really hurt about how you're treating her. From now on, I want you to start noticing what your Inner Bitch is saying and begin to change the language you use when speaking to yourself. Think how you'd say it to a dear friend or a young child. You won't become 'soft' (yes, I feared that too), although you may 'soften' a little into becoming a kinder, more understanding person towards yourself. Another technique that Kristin Neff recommends is to put your hand on your heart as you talk to yourself – a gesture of physical tenderness, even from yourself to yourself, activates the 'care-giving' response in your brain rather than the 'flight-fight-freeze' response. It sounds silly, and it may feel silly at first, but try it. Put your hand on your heart, or on your arm if you're in public, and say something soothing to yourself either out loud or in your mind like, 'Honey, I know you're really worried about this, but we've got through this kind of thing before and it's going to be OK.'[134]

Beating yourself up doesn't work, I can guarantee you;
I did it for years and all I got were bruises.

Healthy self-critique and harsh destructive criticism are very different: one builds confidence and enables us to learn from our mistakes, whilst the other trashes self-esteem and leads to entrenched, repetitive and dysfunctional patterns of maladaptive coping. It's important to learn the difference. For me, I needed to learn how to be kind, loving and accepting towards myself *before* I could 'hear' the difference. These days, I actively seek critique from people whose opinion I trust. I feel that even if I hear something I don't like, I'll be able to handle it and that it will be helpful. I'm also able to make a decision on how to react and act on such information, rather than making a snap judgement such as 'I'm wrong' (which I'd interpret as 'I'm a bad person') or 'They're wrong' (which I'd read as, 'They're trying to hurt me').

Depending on your personality and your childhood experiences with your early carers and teachers, you will have a different 'tone' of Inner Bitch and a different degree of tolerance to criticism. However, learning to be kinder to ourselves is something we can all do and if we want to move forward with our Plan B, it's essential. We need our Inner Bitch on our side by training her to become our Inner Mother – protecting, guiding, teaching, nurturing and gently pointing out areas for improvement rather than yelling at us from the moment we wake up, 'You're useless!'

Self-compassion isn't just an 'idea', it's a set of thinking techniques that change the way we respond to stress. No matter how harsh you are to yourself, you can learn a new way of being. I've come to understand that learning self-compassion is analogous to learning a new language: it takes time and you need to make quite a few mistakes and take a few wrong turns before you get the hang of it. And like a language, self-compassion cannot be learned just by reading about it; you absolutely have to practise it to see the benefits.

I've already described the best two tools for getting started, in my opinion, but here they are again in brief:

- Putting your hand on your heart and giving yourself a soothing pep talk when you're struggling or stressed.

- Monitoring and shifting your internal language from harsh and destructive self-criticism to supportive and self-compassionate constructive critique. And beginning to 'hear' the difference.

Learning to be a 'Good Enough' Mother to Ourselves

The influential twentieth-century English psychoanalyst Donald Winnicott developed the concept of 'the good enough mother': one who was not perfect, but robust enough to allow her child the freedom to explore, and a strong enough sense of safety and security to do so.[135]

For me, this idea of being 'good enough', rather than either perfect or terrible, has been hugely transformational. I used to be an 'all or nothing' person when it came to self-care and found it hard to know the difference between self-care and self-indulgence, or between discipline and neglect. I believe that I probably inherited some of my mother's anxiety around these issues, at her knee and by her example, as she probably did from her own mother.

During my forties I went a long way towards developing a healthier way of relating to my inner world with the help of some excellent therapists, by attending twelve-step groups and through training to become a psychotherapist. Now in my fifties, I have discovered that my capacity for articulating my vulnerability is highly valued by others, as it often encourages them to share *their* most tender spots. My vulnerability and my willingness to talk about it turns out to be one of my greatest gifts, not a weakness at all. *Take that, Inner Bitch!*

Now, before you think, *But I don't have a decade to sort this out!*, I'm not suggesting that you need to do what I've done to get to the place that I'm at because, during my decade of inner work, I gradually put together tools to work with the core distressing issues of childlessness, and also a global network of childless women to support you. Recently, a woman at one of my workshops asked, 'How did you manage to get through this without Gateway Women?' and my answer? 'I nearly didn't.'

I wish Gateway Women had been around when my marriage was ending, although, to be frank, I wasn't ready then – I was still hopeful, still in denial at thirty-eight. It saddens me now to think how different those first few post-divorce years could have been if I had been able to reach acceptance sooner about never having children. But I guess I needed to go through that to get to where I am today, so it feels worth it – and anyway, hindsight is a wonderful thing, and I'm through with *What if . . .*

The result of this work has enabled me to stop seeing myself as 'damaged goods', but rather as a tender-hearted human with the capacity to heal, given the right encouragement and support. Just like you; just like all of us.

Being 'good enough' also means that we give up beating ourselves up when we get being 'good enough' wrong.

For example, I use food to comfort myself when I'm stressed, lonely, tired or upset. I've done it since I was a child – wolfing down whole packets of sweeties in secret. It didn't show up in my weight for years – I was a skinny kid and teenager. As an adult, I gave myself an incredibly hard time about this and went on all manner of diets, gave up food groups and suffered from both undereating and overeating problems. And I got plenty of support from the media for making my body the site of all my problems. I came to see myself as someone who 'had issues with food'. The thing is, I don't anymore; it's a victim identity and I don't feel like one of life's victims now. Instead, I'm aware that food is something that can comfort me and that, within 'good enough' limits, it's not only absolutely fine, it's self-care! I know what my 'good enough' limits are and I stick to them in a 'good enough' way – I don't keep sugary snacks in the house (biscuits 'talk' to me!), but if I feel like some chocolate, I'll buy some and eat it. I've learned to read a desire for something sugary as a desire for some nurturing, so I've also learned to spend some time working out what it is that's creating that need: am I tired? Unwell? Overwhelmed? Lonely? These days I nap when I'm tired; stay in bed when I'm ill; cancel social appointments if I'm overwhelmed; seek out company if I'm lonely.

Sometimes my Inner Bitch wins and I don't nurture myself and instead I get stuck in a self-punishing regime of 'Don't stop, Don't rest, Don't be ill, Don't need anyone.' The fact is, I don't get it right all the time and sometimes I have to fight through a wall of resistance in order to nurture myself. Dealing with being both single and childless along with working from home can sometimes mean that I'm on my own too much – which I have to keep a loving eye on as too much social isolation can be fertile ground for my Inner Bitch.

> *Sometimes there's an internal discussion going where my Inner Bitch and my Inner Mother are arguing. Recently I mislaid my phone and my Inner Bitch said, 'Typical! Just like you to lose your phone, how stupid, all your photos and contacts are on there, you didn't bother to back it up, how can you be so lazy as to not do that?!' and then my Inner Mother piped up with, 'It's OK to feel bad, things like this happen, don't be so hard on yourself. I'm sure it will turn up, and if doesn't, then you have insurance and you can get the photos from friends and family and the contacts can be re-grouped.' They battled it out in my head. Self-compassion won the day, but my Inner Bitch gave her a run for her money!*
>
> Delia: 48, Living with Partner, UK

Each time I substitute a nurturing Inner Mother message for that of my Inner Bitch and discover that, after I've taken the nap, turned down the offer or phoned a friend, that the world is still turning, it gets easier the next time. It's a little bit more data that proves that my Inner Bitch isn't always right. She's entitled to her opinion – after all, she's only trying to look out for me – but it's just an opinion, and a very 'young' one at that.

> *Many of my Inner Bitch beliefs come from around the time I was a teenager, and sometimes I forget that I'm not one anymore. So it's helpful to keep in mind that I can choose whether to listen to her opinion or not.*
>
> Sophia: 50, Single, UK

By taking action like this I am becoming the sort of 'good enough' Inner Mother to myself that I would have been to my own child or to the little 'Russian doll Jody' who lives within me: indulgent (within sensible limits), kind, honest and supportive. And not afraid to point out, with great love, where I might be going wrong sometimes.

Winnicott's work showed that the 'good enough mother' was actually *better* than the 'perfect mother', because a perfect mother (if she existed) would actually stifle our development. For us, being a 'good enough' version of ourselves is all that we need expect of ourselves. Perfectionism is another face of 'not good enough' and another classic platform for the Inner Bitch – a desperate way to maintain an illusion of control in an uncontrollable world.

Give yourself a break. Try showing yourself some kindness and compassion instead of being harsh and judgemental. You'll see that the world doesn't actually fall apart.

It's an illusion that being mean to yourself is the only thing that keeps you 'in check'. You wouldn't expect a child or a puppy to do well with that kind of training, so maybe it's time to take a new approach with your relationship to yourself.

Nurturing the Mother Within

For those of us who wanted to be mothers but for whom it didn't work out, it's important to recognise that our desire to give, to nurture, needs an outlet in our lives. If we *don't* have an outlet for that feeling, it may become 'stuck energy' and may even be what fuels some of the psychodramas we have going on with our Inner Bitch.

I love caring for my chickens and my cat; how they trust me and make me chuckle. Growing up I never thought of being a mother – I never played with dolls, for example – but wanted to live on a

*farm with lots of animals. A few years ago we moved to the country
and so now I get to have all the animals I want. My Inner Bitch
said animals would be a poor substitute for children. But after a
while I told her to shut up, went to the animal rescue and picked
up my cat; then came the chickens. I've always loved animals. They
feed my soul. I feel at ease in nature; it reminds me that I'm a part
of something bigger, something that will continue living after I'm
dead. I thought I needed children for that, but they are not the only
way. Once I saw that, I felt at home in the world again.*

Marjon: 43, Engaged, The Netherlands

It can be hard to know what to do with our nurturing drive, particularly if we don't have a partner and may therefore also be starved of touch and intimate connection. Many of us have pets and this helps a lot, but then some of us deny ourselves that pleasure for fear of becoming the stereotypical childless woman with a cat or dog, whilst others are unable to have a pet for any number of reasons, even though they long to. And then some of us of course really aren't that fussed about pets!

Pets, partners or neither, there is someone we *can* nurture and she's probably in desperate need of it – and that's ourselves. (Oh yes, I felt you pull back from the page then! Stay with me . . .).

It can feel hard even *contemplating* the idea of nurturing ourselves these days as it requires developing an intimacy with ourselves that we may have shut off. We may also have to battle through ideas of 'self-indulgence' and 'self-obsession' before we'll even consider it.

However, for a moment, imagine you were a mother taking care of your child – would that have felt self-indulgent or would it have been loving and thoughtful?

Self-care is a real stumbling block for an enormous number of women; mothers too. I'm not sure what's happened in Western culture that we're bombarded all the time with exhortations to 'take care of ourselves' (which usually requires us to do something to make our bodies look other than they do), yet very few of us seem to really feel comfortable giving ourselves the time to nurture ourselves. Somewhere along the line self-care and self-indulgence seem to have merged ... I sometimes wonder if it's an almost puritanical thing, as it seems to me that women in more Catholic cultures, such as France, Spain and Italy, seem to treat themselves much more generously and kindly and don't seem to feel guilty about it!

Self-care is not self-obsession,
Self-care is not selfishness,
Self-care is not self-indulgence,
Self-care is self-respect.

For me, I've come to understand that self-compassion, self-care and grief work together form the absolute bedrock of my recovery from childlessness. And I suspect that as they continue to develop into my new way of being in the world I will experience a continuing improvement in my sense of internal peace and well-being.

The internal resistance that can come up to these, perhaps new attitudes and techniques, can be huge. I've seen an awful lot of eye-rolling in workshops when I've mentioned self-care, and I've come to understand that sometimes we avoid it because being kind to ourselves can bring up even more grief – although in fact, that's actually more healing ...

EXERCISE 12

The Feel Good Menu

Choose an item to experiment with from each of the four 'courses' on the Feel Good Menu. Some tips:

- Commit to doing one self-care action a day, or a couple per week – whatever you feel you can manage for now. It's important not to set yourself up to fail.

- If there is a 'course' on the menu that strikes you as totally nuts or particularly self-indulgent, that may indicate that this is an area of self-care that you've neglected for some time ...

- If one of the suggestions *really* turns you off, that's probably an activity to choose rather than avoid!

- If there is any terminology in the Feel Good Menu that bugs you, change it to something that doesn't. Don't let that be the reason to skip this exercise.

- Some of these menu items could be listed under a different 'course' – after all, we're complex human beings, not a menu! Don't let your analytical mind get bogged down in the details, that's just a way of resisting doing it.

- Feel free to order off-menu! See the menu items as invitations and ideas to guide you rather than as absolute prescriptions. A wonderful book full of suggestions for every month of the year is Sarah Ban Breathnach's *Romancing the Ordinary: A year of everyday indulgences*.[136]

- Make your own version of the Feel Good Menu and stick it some-where where you'll see it regularly, like the inside of a kitchen cupboard. There's a printable version of it on the Gateway Women website.

- Expect a surprisingly *huge* amount of internal resistance to doing this exercise, but do it anyway.

THE FEEL GOOD MENU

See Appendix for further resources

Heart Course

Hug someone and/or ask for a hug.

*Share how you feel with a trusted, loving, non-judgemental
friend – and ask them to refrain from giving advice unless asked.*

*Be vulnerable – it encourages others to be vulnerable
with you, and creates a healing intimacy. Choose
wisely who you're vulnerable with . . .*

*Sing on your own or yell at the top of your voice. I find this
is wonderful for releasing anger, particularly if I do it in the
middle of a field or somewhere I know no one will hear!*

*Choose to trust yourself. If in doubt, look in
the mirror and ask your own advice.*

*Play with your pet, and if you don't have one,
borrow someone else's.*

*Watch silly clips of cats or dogs on YouTube or
anything that makes you laugh out loud.*

*Call someone that you care about but
haven't spoken to for far too long.*

Watch a film that makes you laugh and/or cry and really let rip!

Spend time with someone in your life who nurtures you.

Head Course

*Talk to yourself as you would to a dear friend or
small child. Give your Inner Bitch the day off.*

*Stop reading women's magazines and practise going a whole
day without beating yourself up about the way you look.*

*Keep a journal or start doing Julia Cameron's 'Morning Pages'
to clean out the mental rubbish.*[137]

*Say 'thank you' and feel gratitude for each part of
your body as you bathe, shower or moisturise.*

Take a deep breath and remind yourself, 'This too shall pass'.

Write a letter to your younger self or your older self.

Make a list of your accomplishments, skills and qualities.

Go on a 'news fast' for a day, a week and then try it for longer.

*Make a list of ten things to be grateful for
every night before bed for a week.*

*Clean out your email inbox and unsubscribe from
all the newsletters and emails that you don't read.
Take a break from social media sites.*

Body Course

Take a nap without setting an alarm clock.

*Cook yourself a healthy and delicious meal and set
the table for yourself as an honoured guest.*

*Soak in a hot bath with a delicious drink, candles, music
and an enjoyable novel. Give yourself permission to
switch off. Don't take the phone into the bathroom!*

Buy yourself some new underwear and get rid of all the 'tired' stuff.

Dance around the living room alone to your favourite music.

Give yourself a pedicure and paint your toenails a wild colour.

*Go swimming, walking or cycling outdoors for at least
fifteen minutes. Or just sit with your face in the sun.*

Walk barefoot on the ground for at least fifteen minutes.

Do some gardening and weeding or tend to your houseplants.

*Declutter your wardrobe and give away all the clothes you
don't wear. Think, 'If this fitted me, would I wear it this
season?' If not, let it go. If that feels too tough, pack them
away in a box, and if you don't need them in the next
three months, give the box away without opening it.*

Source Course

Spend some time alone in nature and leave your phone at home.

*Learn to meditate by taking lessons or listening
to guided meditations. Explore different tools and
techniques until you find the one that's for you.*

*Choose a pack of goddess, angel or archetype cards and pick one
every morning as 'guidance' for your day. This isn't magic; it's
just a way of focusing your thoughts and intentions for the day.*

*Pray in your own way each morning. Say 'thank
you' more often than 'please' – gratitude and joy are
proven to light up the same areas of the brain.*

Think of someone who may be lonely and give them a call.

*Create a 'happiness jar' and try to put at least one note in it each
day to remind you of something good that happened. When you're
feeling blue, or at the end of each year, you can open some/all of
them up and remind yourself of all you have to be grateful for.*

*Find a way to do a secret good turn for
another person every day for a week.*

Listen to a guided visualisation tape or recorded birdsong.

Forgive yourself for your mistakes. Forgive others theirs too.

Visit a sacred place, whatever that means to you.

Reflections on Chapter 9

In this chapter we've begun to explore some of our inner worlds – both our Inner Mother and her shadow, our Inner Bitch. We are all made up of shades of light and dark and indeed, one cannot exist without the other; but for many of us, finding out that we're not the only one that's staging a one-woman campaign against our self-esteem can be a huge relief! It can also come as quite a shock that a 'nice person' like us can be so utterly horrible inside our own heads ...

How has it been for you to look at your inner world in this way? Did you manage to catch your Inner Bitch in the act of destructive criticism, and did you practise shifting your language to something more self-compassionate and supportive?

For many of us, tuning into our harsh inner voice can be extremely illuminating because, perhaps for the first time, we realise that we have more control over how we feel than we thought. However, it can also be a really big shock to realise how much we've been bullying ourselves, and this can bring up feelings of shame. Shame and the Inner Bitch are very closely related.

It's as if we've reached down into some murky water and stirred up the mud at the bottom and things are looking a bit cloudy at the moment. The trick is to skim off some of that muck now before it settles back down again! Although it might be a shock to discover how horrible we've been to ourselves, now we know a bit more about what's going on, we can do something about it. What a relief to know that we're not doomed to feel so awful about ourselves forever!

Sometimes, the resistance we feel to doing something differently, even something that we think we're going to enjoy, can be really strong. It may also bring up some grief and sadness and it might therefore feel easier to put it off for another day. Whether you did or didn't follow through with your intentions with the Feel Good Menu, you may still have found it hard – you may be shocked to realise how long it is since you've focused on doing something that made you feel good, or sad that the prospect of doing so turned out to be much scarier and more emotionally upsetting than you might have predicted. Remember, all change is destabilising to the ego, even the good stuff. So don't give yourself a hard time about it, but choose self-kindness and self-compassion instead.

Self-care, although it looks lovely in the Feel Good Menu and as an 'idea', can actually be very hard to do in practice, and can drive our Inner Bitch nuts, making her step up her messages that we're being 'selfish', 'self-indulgent' and that we 'don't deserve it' or we 'can't' do it until we've done whatever chores *she* decides in that moment are more important! Trying to do your toenails when you've got washing-up to do? Sometimes the noise pollution from the Inner Bitch can make this impossible! If this is, or was, the case for you, use it as a way to really listen to what your Inner Bitch is saying, and imagine you are saying the same words to a friend who wants to spend a little bit of time on self-care ... Hmmm. Sounds a bit harsh, doesn't it?!

'The Feel Good Menu' is not a one-week exercise; it's a lifelong one. Is it worth it? Well, when the prize is getting our mojo back, it definitely is! You've got nothing to lose but your unhappiness, and you can have that back anytime, free of charge.

Transformation sounds like too much effort. I just want to **WAKE UP and GIVE A DAMN** *again.*

CHAPTER 10

Creating a Life for Yourself as a Childless Woman

Why is Creativity Such a Scary Word?
(Terrifying, actually!)

Creativity is one of those words that gets a negative reaction in my workshops faster than almost any other word I know, making some women take a sharp intake of breath and move backwards in their seats! It seems to be one of the best words for making our Inner Bitch jump to attention and say, 'No thank you, we don't do *that* around here!' before you've even had a chance to open your mouth. Yet, as Hugh MacLeod writes, 'Everyone is born creative; everyone is given a box of crayons in kindergarten.'[138]

I've come to believe that creativity is one of the roots of recovery from involuntary childlessness and I also believe that our instant discomfort with the very *notion* of creativity is actually a sign that we're on the right track.

The thing is, we may have become so comfortable with our 'Poor me, I couldn't have children' identity that we're actually a bit reluctant to let go of it. Because, paradoxically, your discomfort has become a place of safety as you're so used to it.

Our ego's job is to keep us safe in an unsafe world and it does a great job of it by making __all__ change seem like a threat. And that includes creativity.

I mean, if we weren't so busy feeling sorry for ourselves and blaming how unimpressed we are with our lives on our childlessness, we might actually have to *do* something about it – and that 'doing something about it' involves change. For those of us who have suffered so much from our dream of motherhood not coming true, dreaming a new dream takes courage. Huge courage with big boots on.

> *I would say that gradually letting go of my fixed identity as a childless woman has been a 'work in progress' over the past couple of years. After some fairly intense grief work, I would describe myself as feeling more like 'me' now, and that I have stepped back into the centre of my life rather than just being on the sidelines. I am a childless woman, and it's part of me that I can take ownership of now, rather than feeling like a lesser person because of it.*
>
> Laura: 47, Single, UK

I have a theory (road-tested to exhaustion in my own life) that we only change when the pain of changing becomes less painful than the pain of *not* changing. And so I can be as stubborn as a mule when it comes to hanging on to things that make me miserable because they feel 'familiar'. I've come to understand that *all* change (even welcome, good change) involves loss, something that has to be let go of in order to move forward. And thus change is hard for almost everyone; but for those of us who've experienced so much loss, we've become almost allergic to it.

Creativity and change are two aspects of the same thing: they're about making something new happen. Bringing into being something that would never have existed had you not been alive. But it brings a side order of loss with it too.

One of the reasons creativity is so scary is that once we take that first step we don't know where we're heading. We're building a new path to a new destination in unknown territory and there's no guarantee that when we get there we're going to like it. When you put it like that, it's hardly surprising that many of us are too scared to take that first step.

But consider this. We've survived worse.

Although we may not know if we can handle anything else 'going wrong', deep down we know that as we've already survived the unthinkable – how bad could it be, really? When I broke up from my first serious post-divorce romance I felt really low. But then I thought to myself, *If I can survive getting divorced from the love of my life, I can survive this ... I'll be OK, eventually. This too shall pass.* (An example of my Inner Mother giving me some kind and pragmatic support.) I'm not asking you to become stoically immune to pain, but instead to recognise that you can be vulnerable, nervous *and* incredibly resilient, all at the same time.

Sometimes, it seems outrageously unfair that not only did we not get to be mothers but that now we *also* have to take responsibility for our own happiness as well. Some booby prize, huh?

But life's not fair – we've learned that. Letting go of that sense of entitlement for an easy life from now on is one of the keys to freeing us up to create our future.

Fed Up with Change

Sometimes when I'm feeling fed up with transformation and the pain of letting go, I get a bit nostalgic for denial. For those days when motherhood was a 'when' ...

I think one of the things that might make us fear change is the idea that 'letting go' of the past means losing it forever, but that's not been my experience. Since that moment on a cold February afternoon when I realised that I would definitely *never* be a mother, I've been in a spin cycle of change. But those changes have not erased my past. Rather, who I was when I wanted to be a mother has integrated with the person I've become, and keep becoming. I have *expanded* my idea of who I am and that includes who I was then. This expansion of my identity has also given me the necessary perspective to be much kinder to the person I was back then. And in turn, that's enabled me to forgive myself for some of the foolish decisions I made (and often blamed others for). I've downgraded my resentment against the world, myself and other people and that's made my reality a lot easier to inhabit.

Giving Birth is Not the Only
Act of Creation

If you accept my definition of creativity as the power to make something exist in the world that wouldn't have existed unless you'd been alive, giving birth to another human being can be seen as the primordial creative act. It's also a creation that keeps evolving and growing and changing.

For millennia, men have both feared and revered women for their power to bring forth life. The entire structure of patriarchy is about putting some kind of ownership boundary around a woman's fertility to ensure that her children are definitely that of the *known* father and therefore able to inherit *his* property.

Giving birth isn't the <u>only</u> creative act. Neither is it the only profoundly energising and meaningful one.

It's important for us as childless women that we find some other way to create – to leave our stamp upon this earth and give birth to something that wouldn't have existed had we not been alive.

I have had to look at my own interpretation of the word 'create' as I do always tend to think of creativity only ever in an artistic way. I now see some of the new projects in my life as creative; for example, I am buying a new home and I have spent the last few weeks putting together some 'mood boards' with ideas for the interior. I'm also thinking 'creatively' about how to develop a new and meaningful working life for myself – something that I have not given any thought to in many years.

Laura: 47, Single, UK

Shadow Artists, Shadow Lives

Julia Cameron, in her influential book about rediscovering our creativity, *The Artist's Way*,[139] writes of the 'shadow artist'. This is someone who longs to express themselves creatively but feels too hemmed in by their fear to do so. So, instead of singing, for example, they work for an opera company; instead of acting, they become an agent; instead of becoming an inspiring public speaker they work as an event organiser. It's as if they want their dreams to keep them warm, but they don't want to get burned. But by getting close, but not quite close enough, after a while they feel frustrated and locked out. Often they then burn out.

For those of us who wanted to be mothers and who live in a world full of other people's children, and maybe even work with them, we too need to be aware of this. We're not going to get to be a mother by the back door and, much as it's (sometimes) wonderful to be around children, forcing ourselves to do so just to prove that we're OK with not having our own may be doing ourselves a real disservice.

> *When I was an elementary teacher, I used to really enjoy being around children, although at times it made my grief even deeper. Now that I feel more 'detached' around them, I suspect it wouldn't be so hard any more.*
>
> Celeste: 39, Single, French Canada

As we get the support we need to do our grief work we may notice that our desire and reactions to being around children change. I went through a stage of finding them adorable, then annoying, then heart-breaking and then I became quite bored with them! These days, it depends on the individual child because I now relate to them as *individuals* rather than as living examples of what I don't have. I'm also OK with feeling annoyed if my peace gets wrecked in an adult-orientated public place like a restaurant. I no longer translate that into *I would have been a terrible mother and that's why it didn't happen.* I just allow myself to feel a bit annoyed whilst also feeling compassion for the parents, who are usually all too aware that their child is being a bit of a pain. I've also found that as I came out of the worst of my grief, I was able to reconnect with the young people in my life in a new way, one based on mutual delight rather than obligation or craving. Those relationships continue to deepen and I feel very blessed to have nephews, nieces, godchildren and other children and young people in my life.

We may not feel nourished by being around children until we have found a way to nourish ourselves.

Until we find that thing that makes our soul sing again, being around children may be a bittersweet experience. But once we've found it we'll be able to connect with them from an authentic place, and they'll feel that too.

I remember when I was about seven or eight and an uncle and aunt of mine came to visit. They always used to bring me such lovely presents, much more thoughtful ones than I was used to getting. However, I also remember that they used to make me nervous as they paid me a level of attention I simply wasn't accustomed to; 'Go outside and play,' was what most adults said to me if I wanted to talk or listen to them. It wasn't until I was a grown-up childless woman myself that I understood that the nervous feeling I had felt around them was probably because they were an involuntarily childless couple. I felt their 'difference' and it bothered me. As a bride, I asked this uncle to give me away in church in place of my father (whom I have never met), not knowing as I did so that I too was destined for a life excluded from the rituals of parenthood. Looking back on it now, I guess it must have been a bittersweet experience for both my uncle, and my aunt watching on.

I've noticed that I find myself moving to a mentoring role with the young women at work who are of an age that they could be my children. When I see babies my heart still contracts, but I do find myself shying away from the under-tens, their noise and their mess!

Natasha: 53, Single, UK

These days, I'm absolutely, genuinely fine with the fact that I don't have children. Some days are easier than others, but occasionally I wonder if I miss the identity and camaraderie of motherhood as much, or more, than having a child in my life. For decades I took for granted the company of my female peers – through schooldays, adolescence, young womanhood and going through my twenties and thirties. And then, over time, as all of them moved to this new place called 'motherhood', I gradually realised that I was increasingly alone – just at the time when it felt like I needed my friends the most. I thought it was just me, but it turns out that this is an experience many childless women experience. It is a cruel irony that childlessness can also involve the loss of a major part of our peer group, as well as the loss of our future family. We are exiled from both our past life and our future life. What our girlfriends, now busy round the clock with motherhood, often fail to realise is that it's rarely just they that are 'too busy' to stay in touch with us – it's most, or sometimes all, of our 'old' friends. It can be very painful for us to see them moving on to new friendships, going on holiday and away for weekends with other families, whilst we struggle to get a date in our diary with them months ahead only to have them cancel at the last minute.

> *My real friends are still real. Those who weren't have moved on, which in hindsight was the best thing that could have happened. A wise woman once said to me, 'How can the flowers in your friendship garden grow if you don't control the weeds?' Oh, how right she was …*
>
> Alizabeth: 41, Married, Australia

Finding Our Creative Selves Again

Some of the world's most well-known female artists are childless or childfree – Frida Kahlo and Georgia O'Keeffe spring to mind – and the single-minded focus of the dedicated artist is often not an easy one to combine with hands-on motherhood. As the English writer, Cyril Connolly, wrote: 'There is no more sombre enemy of good art than the pram in the hall,'[140] and Virginia Woolf, though she longed for children in her marriage, also knew that the role of the 'Angel in the House'[141] (what has now been rebranded the 'domestic goddess') was an all-consuming one that left no room for the identity of the artist.

Having spoken to contemporary female artists who are childfree-by-choice, it seems that they don't feel that they're 'missing out' on something essential by not being mothers because their work fulfils that space in them. They have chosen to put their creative life force into their art, and it shows in their work.

However, this doesn't mean that to find our creative selves we need to all become painters or writers, nor that these activities themselves are some kind of definite path to fulfilment. But rather that there are many ways to live a life that feels meaningful through accessing creativity and embracing our lives again as the lifelong creative project that they are. And there are as many ways to be creative as there are ways to be human.

> *I have taken great comfort and joy from being creative and it has helped me a lot with my grief. I've been busy designing and planting my garden, doing up an old summer house which is now my 'me time' space. Creating something from scratch – making a cake, crocheting a blanket, or making pictures out of shells and pottery picked up from the beach – it's all creative and it wouldn't exist in the world if I hadn't taken the time to create it. It's very satisfying knowing 'I made that'. I have also learned that the things I do don't have to be perfect to be a success, they just have to bring me pleasure in the process – the end project may not win awards, but that's not the point.*
>
> Delia: 48, Living with Partner, UK

I think that a happy, contented 'ordinary' life as a childless woman is a pretty massive achievement in itself – especially when you consider how little support and recognition we currently get from the culture around us, and how hard we can be on ourselves. There is absolutely no need to become any form of Mother Teresa because you're not a mother. Unless that's the sort of thing you would have done anyway ...

Role Models

Exploring the many childless and childfree women role models, both historical and contemporary, has been hugely affirming for me. I've now gathered over five hundred examples as a gallery on Pinterest, with that number growing all the time![142]

It's really important to remember when looking at role models who have a public profile (and are therefore researchable online), that this doesn't mean that *all* childless and childfree women have to do something 'public'!

- **Journalists and campaigners** such as Claudia Jones, the Trinidadian-born journalist who started London's Notting Hill Carnival.

- **Thinkers and healers** such as Claire Bertschinger DBE, the Anglo-Swiss nurse whose work in Ethiopia in 1984 inspired Band Aid.

- **Environmentalists** such as Rachel Carson, whose book *Silent Spring*[143] is credited with starting the global environmental movement.

- **Businesswomen** such as Carly Fiorina, ex-CEO of Hewlett Packard (and US presidential nominee 2016).

- **Children's book authors** such as Tove Jansson and her much beloved 'Moomin' books.

- **Gardeners and cooks** such as perhaps Britain's most well-known cook, Delia Smith.

- **Actresses** such as Maxine Peake, Kim Cattrall, Anjelica Huston.

- **Animal lovers and zoologists** such as Dian Fossey, who worked with mountain gorillas in Rwanda.

- **Adventurers** such as Amelia Earhart, the first female aviator to fly solo across the Atlantic.

- **Musicians and singers** such as Tracy Chapman, Kylie Minogue, PJ Harvey.

- **Politicians** such as Condoleezza Rice (former US Secretary of State) and First Minister of Scotland, Nicola Sturgeon.

- **Dancers** such as the iconic American modern dancer and choreographer Martha Graham.

- **Scientists** such as American theoretical physicist Lisa Randall.

- **Artists** such as 'Young British Artist' Tracey Emin, who has controversially used her abortion and subsequent childlessness as a focus of her art.

> *Living a human life is a creative act in and of itself.*
> *Every moment we make choices that shape our reality*
> *and the environment and relationships around us.*
> *To be alive is to be creative.*

Many of us who have been stuck in grief for years may have parked our creative selves in a side street somewhere, off the main path of life, and might be a bit unsure how to get moving again. We might even feel that it's too late. But it's absolutely *not*, although the process of getting started again can feel a bit daunting – that's our trusty risk-adverse ego again, wanting us to stay 'safe' by staying 'stuck'.

Although it may be painful to observe sometimes, watching children play can remind us that creativity and play are one and the same. Through play, through creativity, children shape their understanding of the world. They take the interior world of their imagination and bring it into the exterior world through their play, and by doing so they form and test their own concepts of how life and reality operate. They are creating the world in their own image, brick by brick, drawing by drawing, game by game. Play is 'work' for children. And that's what we need back in our lives. Although if asked, most people would say that the opposite of play is 'work', the play researcher Dr Stuart Brown has said that, 'The opposite of play is not work. The opposite of play is depression.'[144]

> *It's not just childlessness; being an adult can simply be a shitty experience some days. But it's true that when you are close to children their playfulness can rub off on you. Without kids you can feel that life is an endless set of obligations and tick lists that go on and on.*
>
> Kim: 43, Single, France/UK

The lack of joy, movement and playfulness that so many of us childless women experience as we come to terms with the heavy reality of not having children may possibly be because we are partially stuck in the depression phase of the grief cycle – anhedonia, the inability to feel pleasure, is a symptom of depression.

For me, it seemed an added grief to bear that the things that used to bring me pleasure no longer seemed to have any effect on me. I'd go for a walk in the park to kick through autumn leaves and feel stupid and retreat to the cafe; I'd go swimming, only to find the noise of the public baths deafening and the whole experience cold and unsatisfying. My bicycle stood chained to the railings with flat tyres for years because the pleasure of cycling through London streets and feeling the air on my face had vanished. Those years felt like a kind of death-in-life to me. Not knowing that I was grieving the family I never had, I thought this was just what middle age felt like, and some days I really wondered if I could face an entire life that felt this zombie-like.

In the Gateway Women groups and workshops, I often see similar-looking faces staring back at me as the one I met in the mirror every morning in those years. And when I suggest the idea of play or creativity, of doing something spontaneous, they often look panicked or baffled.

Stuck in grief, in sadness, we forget how to play.
And in doing so, we forget how to live.

We know it, we feel it, but we haven't got a clue what to *do* about it. Everything feels too hard. Or we have the germ of an idea but are too scared to take the next step. It's as if life has turned mean on us and we don't know if we can face any more disappointments when this one, not having children, feels like it nearly wiped us out. Or there again, we take a step towards something playful, something joyful, and our Inner Bitch comes roaring out of the shadows telling us we're 'being ridiculous' or 'wasting our time' and guilt-trips us into backing down and doing the laundry instead – *anything* to keep us away from exploring creativity, which will lead to unpredictable change, and thus risk. And, as many of us know, the Inner Bitch can be brutally effective.

There was no joy in my life for a very long time and it's only
recently that I've felt it again by letting myself become immersed
in creative textile work and ALLOWING myself to feel it! It's been
so hard as guilt seemed to go hand in hand with joy and fun for
me, as though I'm not allowed to have fun. I've had to work very
hard to shake off the feelings of guilt that permeated every aspect
of my life.

Marianne: 63, Married, UK

Illness as a Defence Against Change

When I talk of Plan B, I'm using it as shorthand for a 'life of meaning'.
Plan B is a life that gets you out of bed in the morning and that you feel
excited to talk about when someone asks you about yourself.

Many of us have become defined by our failure to become mothers
and the loss not only of our families, but also of the camaraderie and
belonging of motherhood. Of course, motherhood isn't always rosy
and if we cast our minds back to our *own* childhoods we may recall
the way that the identity of motherhood didn't always sit comfortably
with our own mothers. But losing out on that identity, especially if
we've spent a huge chunk of our life so far hoping and trying to make
it come true, can leave us hollowed out, formless and feeling almost
invisible.

When we look at childfree-by-choice women (and there are all
varieties of them, just as there are all varieties of us, and of mothers)
we might envy them just a little. After all, they *knew* they didn't want
to be mothers, lived in a time when it was possible to make that
choice and got the life they wanted. They're not hollowed-out husks,
invisible, lacking identity. Neither are they necessarily defined by their
childfree status.

Losing the possibility of the mother identity can be so devastating
for us that we may subconsciously want to hang on to it by remaining

stuck in grief. And one way that this might show up as a way of resisting creative living is through illness.

Many of us talk of 'my body' as if it were something separate from us; a fleshy, watery envelope that we inhabit and that does strange things that we don't always agree with. But this is a way of thinking that simultaneously separates us from our bodies whilst also allowing us to avoid taking responsibility for ourselves.

If there's something we don't want to deal with yet, like acknowledging that we need a new idea for our life now that we know we're not going to become mothers, a way of avoiding that can be to develop illnesses. The word 'psychosomatic' is often bandied around like some kind of slightly distasteful neurotic habit, but with it the medical profession acknowledges that the mind is capable of creating physical symptoms that are genuine – that an illness can be, in part, created by the mind. Another of my favourite concepts is the 'placebo effect', in which the ability of the mind to heal the body *without* the intervention of drugs is both expected and allowed for during clinical drug trials. So you see, you don't have to have a dream-catcher on your porch to acknowledge that our minds and bodies work together in ways that are, as yet, little understood by modern medicine, to create both illness and wellness.

Denial, the first stage of the grief process and often the first stage of the change process, is a ripe ground for psychosomatic illness. Whilst I was in the depths of denial about my infertility and the car crash my marriage had become, I came down with every illness going around the office, as well as food poisoning, migraines, tooth abscesses and a binge-eating disorder. I spent the best part of a year too ill to think. Which was exactly what I wanted! I didn't *want to* think. I wasn't ready.

If you are unable to contemplate your Plan B because of an illness, or a series of minor illnesses, it might be worth listening to your body, because it's *definitely* listening to you. It might be that you are forcing yourself to take the next step before you are ready and that what you really need right now is some support with processing your grief. Or it might just be that you're scared of change and being ill gives you a type of solid identity that you're not ready to give up yet. You may also be burned out and in need of a period of profound rest. Once upon a time, we used to have a thing called 'convalescence'. Our need for it at a physical level still exists; it's just that our 24/7 culture doesn't have space for it. We're all meant to be busy 'doing' something – all the time. Sometimes, it seems that the only way to get that kind of rest is to burn out so that we have no other option. It happened to me and I'm now much more alert to the warning signs and let my Inner Mother take charge at that point and not my Inner Bitch!

It's important that you don't think I'm saying that all illness is in your mind and that therefore it's *all your fault*. I am not a medical expert and I'm only drawing from my own and others' experiences that I know of. Many of us are childless because of chronic conditions and I'm not saying that positive thinking or any such woo-woo is going to make ME, MS, cancer, fibromyalgia or any of the other conditions that stop us in our tracks, go away. There is a plague of positive thinking that has come from the US (and which perhaps reaches its apogee in the vernacular of cancer and infertility treatments) that can be oppressive and shaming – *I had a negative thought about my treatment/IVF/recovery chances and that's why it's not working*. Barbara Ehrenreich, the American feminist and social journalist, wrote an excellent book about this – *Smile or Die: How Positive Thinking Fooled America and the World* – having been exposed to the tyranny of such thinking during her own cancer treatment.[145]

So, if you have a chronic condition, please don't add this to your list of things to blame yourself for – it's not going to help. However, if you are ill because you need time to cocoon and this is the only way you know how to give yourself permission to do so, then this is where you need to be. But if you know, deep down, that your cocooning time has passed and that you're stringing it out because you're terrified of taking charge of your life again, then maybe it's time to take a risk with a tiny bit of creativity and see what happens.

You know the answer: trust yourself. And if you're not sure, experiment. Do the exercise at the end of this chapter in the tiniest way you possibly can and see how it makes you feel. Listen to that. Sometimes not becoming a mother can leave us with a profound sense of mistrust in ourselves, so it's hardly surprising that we find it hard to initiate change.

Learning to trust your ability to know what's best for you can be as healing as actually <u>doing</u> what's best for you.

Your relationship with yourself has taken a hell of a battering and there's no shame if you need time to rebuild. After all, blowing up bridges is a lot faster than building them ...

Warning! There Be Dragons

I believe that reconnecting with our creativity and debugging whatever terrors the word brings up for us is an absolutely vital part of not only recovering from our childlessness, but also in creating a life that works for us. And that's what Plan B is all about: creating a new life for ourselves that has meaning, passion and purpose at its core.

What that means for each of us is different. We need to have a conversation with our soul and slay a few dragons too. We need to get off the sidelines of our life, and become our own heroine again.

> *In some ways the 'next' version of me has been a reclamation of the personality and interests I had in my twenties, before the stress of trying to find a partner and have a child kicked in.*
>
> Sarah: 45, Single, USA

Some of those dragons will probably be the people around us who care about us the most. Because creativity equals change, any movement we make towards creativity will probably awaken *their* Inner Bitches and you may hear dispiriting comments such as, 'Yes, but do you really think it's a good idea at your age?' or, 'But how will you find the time?' or some remark that you may have already had to deal with from your own Inner Bitch. Somehow, hearing it from someone else as well can have the unfortunate effect of confirming to you that whatever it is you were planning, no matter how small, is probably a bit ridiculous, a bad idea and maybe even a bit embarrassing. 'Oh, it's just a silly idea I had!' you might find yourself saying ... and you're back where you started. So, my advice is this: when you're getting creative, in however small a way, DON'T SAY ANYTHING. Just do it. And *keep* doing it, and *keep* not saying anything. Once your Inner Bitch has realised that the world's not going to end because you've taken up gardening again or are writing poetry, baking cookies or getting your bike out of the garage, then other people's Inner Bitches won't have the power to shut you down. As Hugh MacLeod writes in his brilliant short book *Ignore Everybody: And 39 Other Keys to Creativity*, 'Great ideas alter the power balance in relationships. That's why great ideas are initially resisted.'[146] If you remember the 'Going Dotty' exercise from Chapter 8, I'd add to that that *any* change, no matter how small, can have the same effect ...

In the next chapter we're going to start constructing your Plan B. It will probably be the first of many because as you grow, heal and change, your needs and desires will change too. We are always a work in progress, just like everything else on earth.

However, with our tendency to be harsh and exacting with ourselves, we may make our first Plan B all work and no play. And that's not going to get you out of bed in the morning, is it? So, this week's exercise is to help awaken your playful side again. Yes, I heard you groaning at the back!

Getting Creative to Find Your Plan B

Grab a pile of Post-it notes or small pieces of paper. Use them to write down individual words or phrases that come to mind in response to this exercise.

1. Write down your answers to the following questions. Do it spontaneously and put down your first thoughts. If nothing comes to mind, move on to the next prompt. Try not to think about it too much, or what your answers might 'mean'.

   - What five words or phrases pop up when you think of the word 'creativity'?

   - What five things or games did you love doing or playing when you were a child?

   - What do you wish you hadn't 'given up' from when you were a child?

   - What adult activity puts you into a place of 'flow'? (Where time seems to soften and you are completely absorbed and at peace.)

2. Now, spread out all your answers (if they are on Post-it notes, stick them on a mirror or window). Jumble them all up. Can you see any patterns or themes emerging? Group them accordingly.

   - Choose a tiny step that you can commit to this week to bring one of these themes alive. It doesn't have to be a huge commitment (that's your Inner Bitch talking) and it *definitely* mustn't be worthy or productive. In fact, the smaller, least complex and more frivolous the better!

   Depending on your personality and abilities, what's fun for you might be hell for someone else, so please don't feel constrained by the following random examples:

- Listen to music that you love and haven't listened to in a while.

- Go to the kind of place you used to enjoy browsing through such as an art gallery, craft centre, museum, tool store, art shop, bookshop, farmers' market, garden centre, junkyard or library – anywhere that inspires or intrigues you, but which you notice you've been avoiding recently. Buy a postcard or some small thing as a memento. Notice what you are drawn to.

- Spend time going through your clothes and wear something that makes you look and feel great – just for the hell of it.

- Declutter your bedroom, rearrange the furniture, give it a good clean and make it feel special again.

- Get your camera out and go for a walk. Photograph anything that catches your attention. Print out the pictures and stick them up or perhaps share them with others in the Gateway Women online community.

- Do some sewing or baking, purely for fun.

- Write a poem.

- Make a cushion or other craft project.

- Drive a new route to work, eat a different lunch, talk to different people.

- Read a biography of a childless woman you admire (if you need some inspiration, take a look at the Gateway Women gallery of childless and childfree role models on Pinterest[147]).

- Plant some new flowers in your garden, buy yourself fresh flowers, get creative with some flower arranging.

- Fix something that's broken with your own hands: the lawn-mower, the computer, the kitchen cupboard, your motorbike – whatever feels like the most *fun*.

- Go horse riding, wild swimming, ice-skating, rock climbing, salsa dancing or karaoke singing – whatever you either used to do or always wished you could do.

Reflections on Chapter 10

In this chapter we've been looking at how our childlessness and creativity are linked, often in surprising ways. These kinds of new thoughts can stir up a lot of old memories and perhaps some more grief. This is not a sign that you are weak or that you are not capable of healing and creativity – in fact, it means exactly the opposite. A healthy psyche will not allow us to experience feelings that we are not yet capable of coping with; that's what denial is for. If you can feel it, you can heal it.

Beginning to look at how other childless and childfree women have chosen to spend their lives other than being mothers can be really challenging at first. It's amazing how our Inner Bitch, instead of being intrigued and inspired by such examples, can use it as yet another reason to put us back in our box, telling us, 'Well, you're never going to be the first woman to fly solo across the Atlantic, so there's no point thinking about going to dance classes again!' or some such illogical (but highly effective) nonsense! Remember, the reason such women are in the Gateway Women role model gallery is because they've done something noteworthy. It absolutely doesn't mean that *your* Plan B has to be 'big' ... So if your Inner Bitch is trying to belittle you because you don't really have a clue about what shape your Plan B might take, take heart that you're not alone wrestling with such dispiriting thoughts. Try writing them down and examining them so you can see how ridiculous some of them are, and ask yourself if you'd ever say any of them to someone else trying to rebuild their life and identity after a devastating loss ...

The notion that you may have developed illnesses as a defence against change can be quite provocative – did it give you pause for thought or did the very concept of it make you furious?! And how about the idea that birth is not the only creative act? Did it give you a surge of hope or perhaps you found it preposterous because the idea that anything could 'replace' motherhood is not something you're ready to give houseroom to yet?

It doesn't matter where you are in your responses to these ideas, but only that you honour where you're at and start from there. Pretending, even to yourself, that you feel other than you do isn't going to move you forward. We've all spent more than enough time pretending that we're more OK with our childlessness than we really are; we don't need to keep up that pretence in private or with other childless women.

How did you respond to the idea that creativity and change are aspects of the same thing? Did it give you some insights into why creativity can feel a bit scary sometimes, or did it perhaps confirm your belief that creativity is just something for 'other people'?

Did you attempt the 'Getting Creative' exercise or was the 'C' word too big for you to deal with at the moment? Sometimes, accessing our playful, creative nature can be quite hard to manage because it may show us how far we've gone from that part of us. Conversely, it can feel *so* good that we feel guilty that we've denied it to ourselves for so long! Then again, it might be that creativity is already an integral part of our life, and so we may begin to wonder whether our passion and commitment to it is one of the reasons we ended up without children ...

Wherever you are is just fine, and the right place for you to be right now. That's what your Inner Mother would say. Turn to her instead of your Inner Bitch and you'll be on your way much faster, whatever the destination!

CHANGE HURTS;
even the good stuff.
Ask the butterfly.

CHAPTER 11

Putting Your Plan B Together

DIY Happiness

Because we don't have children we can't delegate the major part of our happiness, fulfilment and meaning to our role as mothers and our delight in our children – we have to do it for ourselves. And the feedback loop is invisible – no knowing smiles of approval from other parents, no special day in the calendar to tell us how wonderful we are and how much we mean not just to our family, but to the whole world ...

Whilst motherhood is a lifetime of hard work, the results are tangible (even if you don't like them or they bring you great sadness) and once your child is born, usually irreversible. However, creating a life of meaning as a woman without children is a promise to ourselves that no one forces us to keep and which has to be renewed daily. No one's going to take you to court for neglecting *yourself*.

Although as Geoff Dyer, a childfree-by-choice man, provocatively writes in *Out of Sheer Rage*:

> People need to feel that they have been thwarted by circumstances from pursuing the life, which, had they led it, they would not have wanted; whereas the life they really want is a compound of all those thwarting circumstances ... That's why children are so convenient: you have children because you are struggling to get

by as an artist – which is actually what being an artist means – or failing to get on with your career. Then you can persuade yourself that children had prevented you from having this career that had never looked like working out ...[148]

Perhaps, whether you're a mother or not, it's easy to blame your personal circumstances for the reason you are not living your life in a way you feel proud of, when in fact it's part of the human condition to avoid change, as it involves risk. My own feeling is that to steer my life in a way that feels meaningful to me (and to me alone) means walking a very fine line between the needs of my ego (for everything to stay the same so that I'm safe), and the needs of my soul (for adventure and creativity, which involves change and therefore risk!)

I used to fantasise that having children for whom to set a good example would make it easier to 'push' myself, but mothers have helped me understand that this isn't true, and that we *all* struggle with this and find reasons why other things are more 'important' (and less risky). After all, ultimately no one except you can really hold you accountable for making sure that you:

- Write that book.
- Finish decorating so that you're not too embarrassed to invite people round.
- Change your job to one that doesn't make you spend more than you earn in therapy just to cope with it.
- Start your own business.
- Move to the city; or get the hell out of it.
- Stop dressing like your house just burned down.
- Find a way to express your 'mother's heart' in this world.
- Meditate.
- Learn another language.
- Travel up the Amazon.

- Retrain as a garden designer.
- Volunteer at the animal refuge.
- Be kinder to yourself.
- Enter the world chess championship.
- Cook something that doesn't come in a packet.

It's up to us. We get to decide where we're going now. We're reluctant and accidental pioneers in raw new territory; there aren't any maps and precious few roads.

If you feel a little daunted and wonder whether you're up to the job, take heart. I think you'd have to be a risk-hungry adventurer not to feel a *bit* daunted and therefore more likely to be halfway to Alaska by now rather than reading this book!

I often wonder if one of the side effects of becoming a parent is that you realise (probably with a shock) that you are now *definitely* one of the grown-ups. For those of us who are childless we have to take that step alone, invisibly, and, as usual, without anyone encouraging us or giving us a whoop-whoop when we do it. In fact, our families, friends, society and employers often unconsciously treat us as if we are bizarrely aged children compared to our sisters, colleagues and peers who have become mothers.

> *My Plan B has been a series of incremental steps towards feeling OK about how things are. It has been about healing myself from loss, grief and depression, recovering my sense of identity as a woman and as a worthy member of society and about re-growing my self-esteem.*
>
> Hannah: 47, Married, UK

I don't know if you've ever been away from home for an extended period, living in another city perhaps or maybe even another country. The experience changed you, but when you got back, nothing else seemed to have changed and, after a few weeks, everyone forgot that you'd even been away. Being childless and living your Plan B is a bit like that. No one's going to notice much or really be that interested, but we ourselves are changed profoundly, forever.

So, like I said, it's up to us ... and we don't even *have* to do it. There is an alternative: we can always stay where we are for a bit longer, until we're ready. Or we can stay stuck for a lifetime, marinating in a sense of feeling hard done by that harms no one except us. Eventually that gets old. Or we do. The alternative? We can make the best of our lives anyway. No one but us can do it, and no one but us *really* cares. It's not like anyone's ever going to accuse us of being a 'bad mother'. There are no gold stars in life for being a 'good' childless woman, unless you become a saint.

And it's worth remembering that mothers may well have to deal with this stuff later, once their children have left home. But they have a name for it – 'empty nest syndrome' – and get sympathy, empathy, understanding and column inches to help them deal with it.

Debunking Some Plan B Fairy Stories

'Plan B' is another way of saying 'creating a life of meaning' – it just sounds more pragmatic and do-able than 'a life of meaning'. A life of meaning sounds like a bit of a stretch right now, doesn't it?

If you think Plan B is a chance to change your career or get busy so that you don't feel so sad, you're only scratching the surface; this is a chance to create a life that makes you soar. However, before you get too excited by the idea of 'soaring', a word of warning: a fantasy Plan B can be very seductive to us right now. It sounds like the pot of gold at the end of the rainbow; the place where everything is going to be OK, finally; *our* happy ending.

> *For me Plan B represents a meaningful and creative life that is fulfilling. I feel energised, invigorated, and with direction in*

relation to making some major changes in order to achieve this.
I feel that I have taken control of my life rather than just existing
whilst waiting for my life to 'start' (with a husband and children)
– I simply do not have that feeling anymore and my mind feels so
much lighter.

Laura: 47, Single, UK

In the feedback forms filled in after Gateway Women groups and workshops there's often a request for 'more on Plan B, please' and I've created a lot of material around it. But I've come to understand that I'm not really being asked for more material. In some cases the unspoken message is, *Can you please tell me how to sort my life out? I've tried and made a complete mess of it. You seem to have managed it – could you have a go with mine?*

And the answer is this: even if I could, it wouldn't work. It'd be as likely to work out as if I set you up on a blind date. Only you know your heart and soul's desire.

Because, you see, Plan B isn't an idea; it isn't even a plan when all's said and done; it's a process. A process of healing, of growth. And no one can do your healing for you; you can't outsource that.

So What Is a Plan B?

- Creating your Plan B is about having the courage to take risks again when you feel that you've taken enough risks to last a lifetime, and *look* where it got you!

- Creating your Plan B is about learning to trust your instincts and follow your hunches again, despite what your Inner Bitch, your partner, your family, your friends, your boss and the wider world think.

- Creating your Plan B is about finding out who you are again once you drop the 'baby story' and having the faith that there *is* something left, a diamond to be found in the rubble.

- Creating your Plan B is about experimenting with your life and opening up that part of you that dares to dream again, when your last dream nearly killed you.

- Creating your Plan B is about having the self-belief that you deserve to have a happy and meaningful life despite the fact that society, your family and your peers have pretty much given up on you. You damn near gave up on yourself . . .

- Creating your Plan B means making changes to your relationship with yourself, the result of which will cause a ripple of change throughout all your relationships, whether you, or they, like it or not.

- Creating your Plan B means giving up some of the comfortable benefits of being one of life's 'victims' and starting to notice when you're making excuses for yourself.

- Creating your Plan B *also* means learning to be kinder to yourself as a way to encourage your growth and healing and to allow yourself to become the mother to yourself that you would have been to your children.

- Creating your Plan B means thinking about the future, about your old age, about what kind of footprint you want to leave in this world instead of the family you thought you'd have.

- Creating your Plan B is about taking responsibility for yourself and letting go of the idea that someone or something is going to save you. You don't need saving from your childlessness, sorry.

- Creating your Plan B is a radical, line-in-the-sand way of saying to yourself, 'I matter.' Which in turn will start to show up all the things in your life that *aren't* working and which no longer serve you.

- Creating your Plan B is about creativity and change. About dignity and courage. About honouring yourself, standing up for yourself, valuing yourself. It's about paying attention to what matters to you, so that you can offer the best of yourself to your life, and to others.

- Creating your Plan B is about creating a life that fits you from the inside out and learning to accept that others may or may not get that, and that what they think is not actually all that important, frankly!

- Creating your Plan B is about creating a life that, when it's over, you think, 'Well, that was worth it!'

We each have the power, right now, to change the relationship we have with both our past *and* our future. It starts by giving ourselves permission to dream again.

So, if you think Plan B is something that's going to enable you to avoid pain and live an easy life, I'm afraid it's not going to happen. Because nobody gets to have a life like that and, even if you did, you'd be bored out of your mind.

Yes, we may look at other women and think, *Well, her life's a complete picnic*, but we're wrong. *Nobody's* life is free of disappointment, suffering, disease, ageing, loneliness and death. The human condition affects us all. And that includes the desire to compare ourselves to others and feel hard done by.

I realised that I didn't need a Plan B as such, but what I did need was to feel that I had a life of purpose and worth, as well as some self-passion and interest. I have become more like my twenty-year-old self – highly passionate about what it is I believe in and not afraid to speak out. I've also got the benefit of being wiser and more experienced. And I quite like that person ...

Claude: 44, Single, UK

What About the Caterpillar?

The metaphor of a caterpillar becoming a butterfly is often used when talking of transformational change and the story usually focuses on the moment that the butterfly emerges from the chrysalis: this beautiful, elegant creature born from a caterpillar.

But this gets on my nerves. What about the caterpillar? How do you think the caterpillar felt when one day it found itself being entombed in a chrysalis and its entire body started turning to mush? To become a butterfly, the caterpillar has to completely dissolve, right down to the cellular level, and reform. I bet that hurts!

Change hurts, even the good stuff.
Transformation doesn't feel like transformation;
it feels like everything in life has gone to hell and
nothing makes sense any more.

It's only afterwards, when we're out of the chrysalis, that we can look back and say, 'I'm really glad I'm not a caterpillar anymore; that was worth it.' But until then, we have to have a lot of faith that at some point, things will make more sense.

When we were young women we knew that we'd have to make our life 'happen'. We probably spent much of our adolescence and teen-age years mentally and emotionally preparing ourselves for adult life. We thought about how we'd shape the life we wanted and hopefully, mostly, felt up to the challenge. That part of you is still there, and she's smarter than she was when you were young. She's probably also more fearful, but that's wisdom for you.

Whether you're ready to start making changes right now is something only you know. For me, I know that change is on the horizon when I feel utterly and completely frustrated with some aspect of my life and myself; I'm deeply confused and out-of-sorts and I know that I simply *have* to do something about it or I feel I'm going to implode.

But I often don't know what it is I have to do, although somehow I also *do*, I just don't want to admit that I know what it is … It can be a bit messy and often involves tears and a whinge or rant with one of my dear friends, who insists on telling me that it's all going to be fine! I get migraines, backache, avoid phone calls and graze on comfort food. I may even melodramatically resign myself to feeling awful and confused for the rest of my life. When I catch the melodrama soundtrack, I realise that my Inner Bitch is running around and so I talk to myself from my Inner Mother to give myself some soothing and come down from the ceiling!

And then, maybe not immediately, but soon, I realise that something's shifted … Whatever it was that was rumbling below the surface comes into view and is translated into a new thought, new energy, a new decision, a new behaviour, a new insight. My migraine passes, my backache eases and I start eating vegetables again. My good temper returns and I go back to picking up my voicemails.

Because I'm not naturally one of life's great risk-takers, it seems I need to let my frustration (a form of anger) build up a head of steam in order to help me push through my resistance and let the shift happen. I rarely know what the shift *is* until it's underway.

The good news is that I've noticed that this cycle is getting shorter with repetition. I become aware much sooner when the rumbling's started, and offer the balm of self-compassion quickly and regularly. I'd love to say it's now automatic, but it's still a work in progress, and probably always will be! I'm also inclined to be less judgemental about feeling out-of-sorts (thanks to my efforts house-training my dear Inner Bitch!) and much more likely to be curious about what it is that's actually going on, as I know that it means change is coming my way. And I'm not *so* scared of change anymore.

I suspect that one of the side effects of recovering from childlessness is that I trust myself more, and that's making change and taking risks feel less scary. Because these days I trust that whatever happens, I'll cope. After what you've been through, couldn't you say the same? I mean really, how much have you coped with already?

Your Plan B is not a contract with your future self to meet certain goals. It's not a vision board, a bucket list or some worthy resolution. It's a new way of living – a creative way of living – one where you reach out for life rather than sit back and wait for it to disappoint you.

Your Plan B will change over time; it will evolve, as you do. I never thought my Plan B would be to write this book and speak up for child-less women. I thought I was becoming a psychotherapist, but it seems I am also becoming things that I don't even know about yet. Most of all, I'm becoming authentically and unapologetically myself. These days I'm excited to see what I'm capable of and what the future brings, rather than feeling disappointed about what didn't happen. And that's called having your mojo back.

I have made an alternative 'Plan A'; I don't like to think of it as inferior to my first 'Plan A', just different. It is definitely a work in progress, constantly evolving and often surprising. I've realised that the less I try to please others the truer I am to myself and the unique road I am choosing to travel.

Alizabeth: 41, Married, Australia

Follow Your Bliss

So, you get it: no one can tell you what shape your 'life of meaning' is going to have. It's a bit like falling in love – no one can tell you what it's like, only that once you've found it, you'll know.

If I can give you any clues at all, it would be this quote, from the famous mythologist Joseph Campbell: 'Follow Your Bliss.'[149]

I first came across this quote on a greeting card, the year before my marriage broke down. I bought the card to add to the pile I kept in my desk in readiness for people's birthdays and special occasions, but

I found that I could never bring myself to send it to anyone. Instead, I pinned it above my desk and it followed me around in the years following my divorce, always pinned where I was writing (or trying to write). It seemed to hold some essential truth that I was attempting to grasp, but couldn't quite 'get'.

Looking back now, I realise that for a long time the reason I wasn't able to follow my bliss was because I didn't have any to follow. I was dead inside and it seemed that I'd felt that way for so long that I really didn't expect it to change. My life felt finished and I seriously wondered how I would find the energy to keep going. I felt like the 'other' bunny in the Duracell bunny adverts, the one *without* the long-lasting batteries.

But the little Jody (aged about six) who lives on as a Russian doll inside me – the one who used to write stories to read to the fairies in the woods; the one who lay on her back in cornfields and marvelled at the universe spinning around her – she was alive and well. She was the one who knew what that postcard meant and she was the one that hung onto it and kept sticking it above my desk. *She* knew what bliss was, which meant that somewhere I did too. I didn't need to learn it; rather I needed to *unlearn* a whole load of other crap that had got in the way.

The last time I remember seeing that card was around the time that I came out of denial about my childlessness and began thinking, *Now what?* Some of my first Plan B ideas (although I didn't call them that then) were actually part of my grief work and weren't at all about bliss. For example, I seriously contemplated getting rid of all my possessions and moving to Laos to spend the rest of my life living and working in an orphanage on the Mekong River. (I blame *The King and I*!) However, looking back on it now, I can see that parcelled up in that plan was a mixture of romanticised tragic glamour, an escape from the reality of my pain and a desire to have my loss witnessed and understood by others through heroic self-sacrifice. I didn't think much about the orphans at all and it certainly wasn't about following my bliss; it was about following my pain.

My Plan B is to work professionally in an artistic field and to learn the new skills necessary to develop my potential. I have degrees in art but have never been able to accept who I am, choosing to identify myself as a 'childless woman' as opposed to an 'artist'. It feels unfamiliar and scary, but the desire for a better life will get me there.

Marianne: 63, Married, UK

Joseph Campbell said, 'If you follow your bliss, you put yourself on a kind of track that has been there all the while, waiting for you, and the life that you ought to be living is the one you are living.'[150]

The Meaning Map

Having worked with many childless women individually, in groups, workshops and online, it seems that for many of us, thinking about the idea of 'meaning' feels really challenging. I wonder whether this is tied into the motherhood myth that 'being a mother is the most meaningful thing you can ever do', which, if you buy into it, makes everything else a runner-up prize. If you're still of that mindset, I suggest taking a look again at Chapter 3.

A life of meaning will look and feel different to each of us, which is why I can't give you a sealed envelope with your Plan B inside, which is what a participant on one of my retreats admitted she was secretly hoping for! Because, perhaps privately, deep down, sometimes we'd all like it if someone else could just give us the answer to something we're really struggling with. I think that's why I always loved the ending of Douglas Adam's *The Hitchhiker's Guide to the Galaxy* when it turns out that, 'The answer to the ultimate question of life, the universe and everything is 42'![151] Somewhere, it's part of being human to want solid answers to really difficult, often unanswerable questions. And working out your own path to a life of meaning is one of them.

I created the Meaning Map to show some of the different areas of life that are necessary to physical, mental and emotional health, and which can contribute to a life of meaning. It bears some resemblance to other models, including Maslow's famous 'Hierarchy of Needs',[152] Tony Robbins' '6 Human Needs'[153] and the Feeling and Needs Inventory of Non-Violent Communication,[154] but by creating it as a circle, instead of a hierarchical pyramid or list, I find it gives more of a sense of a dynamic system of flowing and interconnecting factors. As many of us who are childless know, following a set of socially prescribed steps to arrive at a predictable plan often doesn't work, and can leave us feeling short-changed by life's 'rules', as we saw them. We can also lose a lot of confidence in our ability to shape our own lives at all . . .

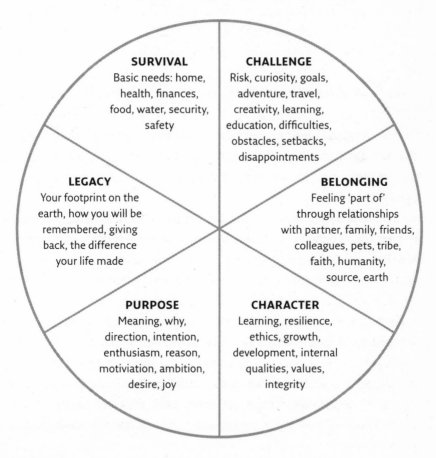

SURVIVAL
Basic needs: home, health, finances, food, water, security, safety

CHALLENGE
Risk, curiosity, goals, adventure, travel, creativity, learning, education, difficulties, obstacles, setbacks, disappointments

LEGACY
Your footprint on the earth, how you will be remembered, giving back, the difference your life made

BELONGING
Feeling 'part of' through relationships with partner, family, friends, colleagues, pets, tribe, faith, humanity, source, earth

PURPOSE
Meaning, why, direction, intention, enthusiasm, reason, motiviation, ambition, desire, joy

CHARACTER
Learning, resilience, ethics, growth, development, internal qualities, values, integrity

If you're averse to the idea that a model could be any help at all with understanding your life, these words from the mathematician George Box illuminate a great truth, namely that, 'all models are wrong, but some are useful'.[155] A model is purely an intellectual way to simplify complexity so that we have an easier time extracting meaning from it. It's not 'the truth', just as a map is not the territory.

If you imagine each of these segments as an area in your life, you will notice that some of them are Survival-level needs, such as a home, food and water, and finances, whereas others are more internal, such as Purpose and Character. We'll be looking at these in more depth in the exercises that follow, but you might like to start thinking about how your life today would 'map' onto this model, to see where your energy is going, and where you might need to divert some of the flow in order to create your own life of meaning.

Being Ready to Look at Your Plan B

It takes great courage to start dreaming again after all we've been through. It's quite likely that we've become overly serious about life and may have lost contact, to some degree, with that playful part of us that used to daydream when we were young. Therefore, before we start our first Plan B exercise, we need to limber up a bit. If, when you read through the following exercises, you think they're a bit trivial, that's probably your Inner Bitch talking and it probably means that they're just what you need ...

> *Initially I was very angry about having to have a Plan B. I want-*
> *ed my Plan A and was not ready to accept that I could be happy*
> *with a different life to the one I wanted. My Plan B is not just one*
> *thing, it's not a business plan or a career change. Plan B for me*
> *means living my life rather than just existing. It means taking*
> *opportunities (and taking some risks). It means participating, and*
> *not sitting on the sidelines. I spent so many years living inside*

my head that I became disconnected from pretty much everything around me.

Heather: 40, Married, UK

It's absolutely understandable that allowing yourself to dream once more, to be playful again, to trust that despite your sadness life will turn out OK after all, is a lot to ask of yourself after what you've been through. But it's not going to magically 'go away' on its own.

We don't get given a new life; we have to create it.

If you've been struggling with the grief of childlessness for years, you may find these exercises very hard, but I'd like to encourage you to have a go anyway. Sometimes, women in my groups and work-shops find it almost impossible to write anything, find the instructions incomprehensible and the whole thing a bit of a mystery and maybe one that makes them furious as well. If this is you, don't panic. What it *may* point to is that you're not quite ready to imagine your future yet, and what might be called for first is a bit more grief work. There's no shame in that, so please don't feel bad about it. Try to do these exercises anyway, and also commit to incorporating more grief work activities into your life. (See Chapter 4 for more information and ideas.) You might find that when you return to these exercises at a later date, something has shifted for you and they feel easier. That in itself can be a great boost to your morale.

In a way I would love not to have to find a Plan B. But I cannot stay where I am – it is too painful. There is only so much loss that you can take before you have to ask yourself what you can build in the world that would make a difference.

Margot: 67, Married, USA

Time Travel

Grab a pile of Post-it notes or small pieces of paper. Use them to write down individual words or phrases that come to mind in response to this exercise.

Imagine you are eighty years old and are looking back over your life. Allow yourself to daydream about the things that are going to happen between now and then *as well as* what has already happened. The only thing you cannot change in the future is not becoming a biological mother.

- **Achievements:** List the ten things that you are most proud of, including those things you hope or anticipate you *might* be proud of by the time you are eighty.

- **Regrets:** Now, list ten things you regret – those things you wish you'd done differently, or which you *anticipate* or *fear* you might regret by the time you are eighty.

Arrange all your achievements and regrets into two separate columns. (Stick them on a window or mirror if possible.) Stand back, and see if you can see any themes emerging.

Can you perhaps see how they relate to the Meaning Map? If you group them into the six different segment areas, can you see that perhaps some segments require your attention more than others?

You may see that some of your themes straddle more than one segment on the Meaning Map, for example:

- If one of your themes is something like 'doing well in my career', this might satisfy your Survival needs through financial security, may Challenge you to achieve your potential and may also contribute to your desire for Legacy if in doing so you are making a lasting difference.

- Or 'creating a beautiful home' might be part of your need for Security as well as for Belonging.

- 'Travel' could be part of your need for Challenge, Belonging and Character.

I very much doubt that any two women's Meaning Maps would look alike, so it's important to know that whatever you take from this exercise is probably unique to you. Because only you will know what sense this makes to you, and what insights you gain from it. There are no right or wrong answers to this exercise; it's just a way to start loosening up your thinking about what's important to you and getting some perspective on that.

So now we're going to let your Inner Bitch have *her* say on the matter of your 'fancy ideas' about meaning!

EXERCISE 15
Uncovering Your Resistance

Grab a pile of Post-it notes or small pieces of paper. Use them to write down individual words or phrases that come to mind in response to this exercise.

Try and write at least ten answers to each question below, and don't be concerned if the same responses come up more than once.

Write down all your reasons, rationales, fears or negative thoughts about:

- Why you *haven't* done more of the things your older self is proud of.

- Why you *can't* do more of the things your older self wished you'd done more of.

- In a nutshell, what *has* stopped you in the past and what *will* stop you in the future?

When we do these exercises in the Gateway Women groups and workshops, most women find their list of 'achievements' as much fun as pulling teeth, whilst their 'regrets' (even the ones that haven't happened yet) are much easier to identify. And as for the things that *have* and *will* get in their way ... frankly it's hard to stop them writing! The answers that they usually come up with are a variation on the following. Do yours fit under these same four categories?

1. **Fear**, including, amongst many varieties:
- Fear of not being good enough.
- Fear of rejection, getting hurt, making a fool of myself.
- Procrastination, indecisiveness, inertia.
- Fear of failure.
- Fear of success.
- Fear of loneliness.

2. **Internal Resources**, including:
- Low self-esteem, not good enough.
- Lack of motivation, lazy.
- Don't know how, not smart enough, too stupid.
- Lack of self-belief, don't deserve it.
- Naturally inhibited, too shy.
- Jealousy, envy, inadequacy, depression, grief.

3. **External Resources**, including:
- Poor health.
- Lack of opportunities, bad luck.
- Not enough support.

- Not enough time, too late, too old.
- Lack of knowledge, lack of talent.
- No time, money or energy left after work.

4. **Other People**, including:

- My partner/parents/family won't like it.
- I'll be judged by others.
- Wanting to conform.
- Being in the wrong relationship.
- Listening to the wrong people.
- Poor parenting means I can't do it.

When I get everyone to put their Post-it notes up on the wall together and ask them to try and group them into categories (I don't tell them the 'titles' of the four categories beforehand), Fear, Internal Resources, External Resources and Other People have so far always shown up. And the one with the longest list has *always* been Fear.

These are women who have usually never met before, of different ages and from different backgrounds. Each of them sees, in front of their own eyes, that what they *thought* were their very own private weaknesses and failings are shared by everyone else in the room.

Our Inner Bitch would have us believe that the reason we didn't get the life we wanted and <u>won't</u> get the life we want is because we're uniquely useless. <u>It's not true</u>.

What we're seeing here is universal; it's called the human condition. Different cultures may have slightly different versions of it, couched in slightly different language, but this stuff, what Steven Pressfield calls 'resistance',[156] is what *all* normal, well-adjusted individuals have to deal with. Despite what we believe, we have not been *personally* singled out by fate to be fearful, worried about what others think, afraid to grasp new opportunities and unsure of our abilities to perform. It's normal.

Like everything else in the universe we are a combination of expansion and collapse; of growth and decline; of forward and back; of love and fear.

Inside, we are all lovable and we are all scared. The trick is to know that everyone, no matter how successful or fearless they seem to you, feels the same inside.

It's time you gave yourself a break for being human. Because once you do, all the energy that went into telling yourself you're uniquely built to fail can go towards creating your Plan B instead.

Beware the Pressure to Be Extraordinary

I want to point out something very important about *who* and *what* your Plan B is for.

Your Plan B is for <u>you</u>. It's about what a meaningful and fulfilling life <u>looks and feels like to you</u>. Not to anyone else.

There is a subtle pressure that because we are childless we have the space in our life to do something extraordinary. But the fact is, we don't have anything to 'make up for' because we haven't had children. That's just more shame talking. But it's a hard one to spot and an even harder one to resist sometimes. I call it the 'Mother Teresa' complex.

It's very easy for us to fall into the trap of thinking that we should be doing something extraordinary with our life. Yet, if you had been a mother, would anyone (including you) have expected such things of you? Why should you have to be Mother Teresa just because you don't have children? And indeed, why shouldn't mothers be allowed big dreams and goals too?

I see my Plan B as a series of smaller changes that ideally I would like to look back on in, say, five years and realise that because they were all interwoven, together they would look like a fairly big change.

Laura: 47, Single, UK

This is another form of the 'not good enough' refrain of shame that comes with the territory of being childless in our culture right now and it's important that you question it. It's a place where your Inner Bitch can take up residence, pushing you forward into projects and places that *look* meaningful but which are actually just more ways for you to prove to yourself and to others that you matter, *even though you're not a mother.*

This is subtle stuff that can hide away from our awareness quite cunningly, so here are a few questions to ask yourself:

- If the results from doing this were invisible, could I be bothered to do it?
- Would I do it even if I didn't get paid for it?
- Would I do it even if no one ever knew about it?
- Who am I doing it for?

Whilst the idea of 'meaning' can seem like a lifebuoy in the stormy seas of childlessness, you don't need to make a grab for every flotation device that comes into view; you just need the one with *your* name on. And finding that 'one' may require some experimentation. It may be that you need to do a few 'big' things before you work out that you don't have the energy for them and that they're just not for you. That's not failure; that's feedback.

> **You don't need a big life on the outside to be a happily childless woman; but you <u>do</u> need a big life on the <u>inside</u>.**

Being a childless woman in our currently motherhood-crazy world can feel like as much of a full-time job as being a mother. It's just that the work is internal, invisible and involves a steady pushing back against the deluge of messages that there's something wrong with us, that we're not welcome, that we've failed. Not being crushed and deformed by those messages, that is *our* life's work. And we'll possibly get no credit from others for it. As a result, we often don't even give ourselves credit for it.

> *Believing I am worthwhile and filling my life with things that are important to me has definitely helped me to live a big life on the inside. At times I do stumble, but I always get up; I owe it to myself.*
>
> Alizabeth: 41, Married, Australia

Whether your Plan B ends up looking ordinary, extraordinary or maybe a bit of both is up to you. It's about whatever kind of love affair with life works for you.

> **We are reluctant pioneers. We didn't choose to be so different, but now that we are, we have the chance to shape and create a life that feels meaningful to us. And to us alone.**

Your First Plan B

Turn off the phone, lock the door, turn off the radio, feed the cat – do whatever you need to get total peace and privacy for about an hour.

Get yourself some paper and pens, or a special notebook. Create a template of the Meaning Map using the instructions from earlier in the chapter or download one from the Gateway Women website. If you enjoy drawing and doodling, get your drawing stuff out. Hell, get the glitter pens, Post-it notes, scissors, fluffy pompoms and gold stars out! (When I do a similar exercise in workshops, everyone looks very nervous when I get such things out, yet by the end, everyone gets into it and a lot of fun is had.) You'll also need a timer. Maybe get yourself something nice to drink and perhaps light a candle. This is meant to be enjoyable so gather whatever you need to make it special for you.

Sit down on a chair, or on the floor, in the garden – wherever you are most comfortable – and spend a couple of minutes breathing gently and relaxing. When you are peaceful and comfortable, set the timer for ten minutes. You're going to do a visualisation exercise.

Close your eyes and imagine a day in your life about five years hence, when your Plan B is moving ahead and you're living a life of meaning, purpose and connection. You're happy and fulfilled and no longer crushed by your childlessness. Life has worked out amazingly well, all things considered, and you can't quite believe your luck.

Let yourself daydream about this day, as if it were happening today. Be playful – this is a daydream after all. Imagine how you'd feel, look, be, behave ...

- What clothes are you wearing?
- What's happening in your life that day?
- What will already have taken place and be in your life on that day?
- What kind of people are around you?

- What is your environment like?
- What does it look like, smell like, feel like, sound like?
- Look off into the distance – what can you see?

Let yourself daydream like you did when you were a child and allow yourself to drift away into this new place ...

And then, when the timer goes off, capture it, in whatever way feels most natural to you:

- Quickly write it all down. Write it in the present tense, as if it were happening today, right now. And whatever you do, don't edit anything out as being stupid or impossible. Not yet. This is play.
- If it's easier for you, or as an experiment, you might want to talk it all into the speech recorder function on your phone if you have one.
- Have a go at drawing what you've seen – that's where the glitter pens come in! Remember this is play and no one needs to see this but you.

Once you feel you've captured it, see if you can map your vision onto the Meaning Map and see how different parts of it satisfy different areas.

This is still fantasy, try not to let your sensible head start editing yet ...

Starting really, really small, for now, choose one element of your vision to put into action. Tiny steps, that's the idea. It needs to be an element that has a positive charge for you, something that gives you a sweet flutter inside that's somewhere between fear and excitement. Nothing worthy or sensible – for example, if losing weight or getting a new job have been on your to-do list for ages this isn't what you're looking for. However, if in your visualisation you were accepting an award for garden design and you love gardening but have never thought you could make a living from it, that's something with a 'positive charge'.

Now, before you start yelling at me that it's not realistic, not possible, can't afford it, what kind of crazy-arsed book is this ... STOP!! *I'm not saying go and do it!* I'm asking you to let yourself have a daydream.

Your first Plan B is <u>not</u> about committing yourself to a course of action that's going to last the rest of your life.

It's not about selling your house, buying a VW camper van and moving to Nova Scotia to study rare birds. In fact, I strongly recommend that you *avoid* doing anything you can't change your mind about. Tiny steps, remember – not *huge* decisions.

What did you want to be when you grew up? A ballerina, a spy, a vet, a nurse, a pop star, a doctor, an explorer? Do you still want to? Probably not. You had other dreams that came later. And so it'll be with your first Plan B. The fact is you're probably out of practice with imagining new possibilities, so I recommend that you keep your training wheels on for a while. Try out a few low-risk ideas and, as your 'sad childless woman' identity starts to evolve into something new, your Plan B will evolve along with it.

So, what's the lowest risk, most fun (it has to be fun!) thing you can do in the next week to try out an element of your daydream Plan B? Go do it.

It can be whatever tickles your fancy:

- Walking through the doors of the art college you've been going past on your way to work and wishing you'd gone there twenty years ago – just to smell the air and pick up a prospectus.
- Writing a poem about looking for your Plan B.
- Finding your sewing machine under the pile of must-do mending and making something just for fun.
- Going beach-combing as part of a garden project, or maybe because you have a hankering to become a geologist . . .
- Signing up for the open evening at your local choir because you used to love singing.
- Heading to the zoo with your sketchbook.
- Cooking a new recipe for that cake shop you fantasise about.
- Doing some hula-hooping, roller-skating, ice-skating – anything

that feels like fun and that you don't do because you don't have kids.

- Getting creative with your wardrobe again.
- And there's nothing wrong with researching whether there *are* any campervans for sale and what qualifications you *might* need to work as a rare breed conservationist specialising in eagles. As long as you actually also *do* something, like going bird-watching.

You just have to take that first tiny step. It all starts with that first step. Self-esteem is built by keeping our promises to ourselves so it's really important that you follow through. Which is why it's also really important to make it genuinely something you really want to do, not too difficult or expensive and definitely not too sensible.

Your Plan B starts when you do, and where might it end up? Who knows? It's an adventure, *your* adventure. Which is good, because on their deathbed nobody wishes they'd spent more time at the office.

Reflections on Chapter 11

In this chapter, we've been looking at creating some of the elements that might become part of your first Plan B – your first tiny steps towards creating a meaningful and fulfilling future without children. Ultimately, it doesn't matter what your Plan B is – it's whatever works for you. One woman's life of meaning is another woman's 'Meh!'.

Although you may have initially been a bit disappointed that I didn't solve your Plan B dilemma, I also hope that you understand that no answer I could give you would ever really wash. That only *you* know what makes your wings itch to fly again, only *you* have the skills to make it happen. And also, that you might need to regrow your wings a bit more before they'll even start 'itching'. This isn't an overnight job.

I hope that the exercise 'Uncovering Your Resistance' gave you some comfort, and that finding out that the things that hold you back are the same for everyone else might encourage you to give your Inner Bitch the day off. Of course, you might find that you use this as further fuel to beat yourself up, by saying, 'If everyone feels this, and other people manage to sort their lives out, why can't I?' Firstly, it's important not to 'compare your insides with other people's outsides', as they say in twelve-step programmes – you have no idea what *so-and-so* actually thinks and feels about themselves. And secondly, thoughts like these may mean that your Inner Bitch has woken up to the fact that you're thinking about initiating some change, which signifies that you're already on your way!

Did you find time to follow through on your tiny step or did you find reasons not to? Sometimes, taking that first step can be surprisingly hard, so if you found it difficult, it might be that it just wasn't fun enough. You may have given yourself something else to add to your to-do list – and that won't do at all! This first step needs to be something you're absolutely busting to do, if only you'd let yourself do it. To get your Plan B going, you're going to need to learn to start experimenting with your life again, so don't see this as a failure, but as feedback to help guide you as you learn what lights your fire.

And if you *did* take that tiny step, how was it? Was it as hard as you thought it was going to be, or was it actually a bit too easy? Perhaps now you've taken that step, you're ready to take a slightly bigger one. This is the beginning of a journey back to ourselves and sometimes it's easier than we think; we just need to give ourselves permission and to seek out and allow some encouragement. We need our tribe.

Although we are now coming towards the end of this book, you stand at the threshold of a whole new beginning. Take a moment to acknowledge how far you've come and make some plans to celebrate when you get to the end of Chapter 12. We have so few rituals as childless women, separated as we are from those of family life, so get together with other childless women and have a ball!

You are
NOT ALONE
anymore.
WELCOME
to your tribe.

CHAPTER 12

Taking Off the Invisibility Cloak

Welcome to Your Tribe

My first thought when I found out that one in five women were turning forty-five without having had children was this: *Well, where the hell are they all then?!*

> *Meeting other childless women like me through Gateway Women has given me so much strength and a sense of belonging to something powerful, wonderful, supportive and full of empathy. Some I've met in workshops, others through Meetups for a coffee and chat. It's a breath of fresh air and great to talk about all sorts of things and know that we all 'get' each other.*
>
> Delia: 48, Living with Partner, UK

Before I started Gateway Women I was, amongst all my friends and colleagues over the years, as far as I know, the only woman who wanted a child and didn't get to have one. I knew a couple of childfree women who'd chosen not have children, but none who'd longed for motherhood and had had to come to terms with childlessness. I felt so isolated in my situation, like I was the only one.

I've spoken to enough childless women now to know that my isolation is quite a common experience. After all, if four out of five women are mothers, the chances of being the only one who's childless in your family and social group must be quite high.

Going to meet other childless women made me a little nervous, but I was also very curious about the others. They turned out to be quite normal people! I wonder where all the childless people are hiding since I never see them in any situation? Are they so ashamed of themselves? Are others ashamed of us? I think we need to educate our society so that we can live our lives more openly.

Liska: 44, Married, Sweden

Amongst those friends several years younger than me and born in the 1970s, however, there seem to be many more who increasingly worry that motherhood isn't going to happen for them. And all of them for reasons of 'social infertility' – in that they have been unable so far to find a suitable partner to raise a family with, and time is running out. Very few of them either want or can afford to become 'solo mothers' by choice. This is increasingly the case for the 1970s cohort joining the Gateway Women online community.

As well as consciously spending more time with my friends who don't have children, I have deliberately cultivated friendships in spaces where I know there are lots of people who don't have children, for example, hiking clubs, Meetup groups and the Gateway Women Meetup here in Dublin. I think it's helped me to have a peer network who are at a similar life stage to me.

Eimear: 44, Single, Ireland

If you turn on the TV, watch movies, follow celebrity gossip, read women's magazines or pay attention to how products aimed at women are marketed, you wouldn't think there was any woman alive who wasn't dating, engaged, trying to conceive, pregnant, married, a mother or a grandmother. And as for women without children over the age of forty, we're almost completely absent from any kind of cultural representation. In academic terms there's a name for when a group is missing from a culture's representation of itself: it's called 'symbolic annihilation'.[157]

Now, I don't know about you, but I haven't been through what I've been through to become invisible!

Accounts of life without children are almost completely absent in our media. There is so much information and support on the issues of parenting and there is significant positive reinforcement and valuing of women who are parents. I think this is a good thing, but I also think that it reflects the needs of the majority and ignores the considerable minority of women who don't have children. In addition to this, the lack of visibility of women who don't have children and the cultural devaluing of alternatives to parenting and the contributions that childless women make are also problematic.

Eimear: 44, Single, Ireland

We looked earlier at some of the cultural reasons as to *why* society historically hasn't been comfortable about mature women without children, but what feels important to me now is thinking about what we can do to *change* that; how we can take our rightful place in society in such a way that it's comfortable for us individually and something that others feel comfortable with too. The fact is, as a group, we have a great deal to offer to our communities, our culture and the wider world. However, before we can get others to realise this we first need to realise it *ourselves*. Each one of us that reclaims our self-esteem and lives a life of meaning (as we understand it) makes a difference. We don't have to rush to the barricades; just living our lives unapologetically and publicly is all that's needed – just as gay men and women have learned to do.

Some of the reasons each of us are needed to show up in the world are:

- **We are leaders:** We can be a huge force for good in this world. Within our communities, businesses and culture there is a tremendous desire for a new, more collaborative way of doing things, and we could be a big part of that.

- **We are role models:** We are women whose hearts have been broken by life but who have had the courage to heal ourselves and move forward. That makes us fabulous role models to those around us personally, to the younger generation, at work and in the wider world.

- **We are guides:** We are deeply compassionate women who are not afraid to support others in their distress and confusion. We may be needed to support our society (most of which remains in profound and fearful denial) through the disruptive transitions ahead as it transitions to a sustainable post-industrial one and grapples with the consequences of climate change. We know that good can come out of even the most dark-looking times.

- **We are wise women:** We are brave, independent, educated, aware, soulful, compassionate women who just happen not to have children. We are that 'village' that is often mentioned that a child needs, so perhaps it's time to break down the ghetto of the nuclear family and find ways to share around the love, and the work, of child-rearing in ways that work for parents, children and us.

- **We are trailblazers:** We are part of the first ever generation of women to be ageing without children in such numbers whilst also being educated and liberated, and we are not in denial about the challenges that come with it. Individually and collectively we can come together to find new solutions. As long as people are too afraid to talk and act on this issue, somehow hoping it'll 'go away' or 'someone else' (often their children) will deal with it, creative solutions are suppressed.

- **We are nomos (the not-mothers):** Individually we're impressive. Collectively, we're awesome.

It's time we removed the invisibility cloak and showed the world what we're made of. Stereotypes can be changed, one woman at a time.

Imagine how different it would have been for you if you had known of *other* women who'd come to terms with their childlessness and had gone on to create a life of meaning? Imagine if such women were a part of our culture – seen on TV and in magazines as normal people, not as cautionary tales or freaks, but just as another way to be an adult woman? Just imagine that for a moment. Let it sink in. Think how much easier it would have been ...

If women without children were to throw off their mantle of shame, they would finally make themselves visible and be able to laugh at everything thrown at them. I wouldn't expect just 'loving' women from this change at all; I'd expect powerful, rebellious, ironic, sarcastic women too, turning the world upside down. If we simply make it as normal not to have children as it is to have them, I think this is the way to go. I kind of like silent revolutions, but first and foremost, things have to change in the heads of those for whom the change matters. And I think there's still a lot of work to do there.

Ada: 38, Living with Partner, Germany/USA

Each one of us who has the courage to feel OK
*about ourselves, despite the messages we're getting
from our culture, is a heroine. We don't need to
be Mother Teresa or Oprah to do this. Just being
ourselves and refusing to feel ashamed is all that
we need to do to start changing things.*

It may be simple, but it won't be easy. As nomo role model Gloria Steinem wrote in 1971:

Any woman who chooses to behave like a full human being should be warned that the armies of the status quo will treat her as something of a dirty joke. That's their natural and first weapon. She will need her sisterhood.[158]

Building Your Tribe

Finding a way to be with other childless women who are exploring, embracing or living their Plan B is just about the best thing you can do to make yourself feel visible again. It's transformed my life and I love watching the process of transformation happen for other women too, whether in the Gateway Women online community or in person.

I decided to make new childless friends as soon as I stopped my IVF journey. I needed to move on and I needed to surround myself with others who understood. Finding an online community where I felt comfortable, accepted and supported was invaluable. Very quickly I transitioned from needing support to offering support. That was a wonderful feeling.

Alizabeth: 41, Married, Australia

In my workshops and courses I see women arrive tightly buttoned up, nervous and shaky, sitting as near to the door as possible, ready to bolt at any minute. Gradually I see them soften and open as the session unfolds. I see a look somewhere between disbelief and relief on their faces as they hear parts of their *own* story coming out of *other* women's mouths. I watch them gradually let go of their fear about being open as they realise, perhaps for the first time, that no one's going to say, 'It's OK, you've still got loads of time,' or, 'You could still adopt,' or, 'Women of fifty are having babies now,' or any of the other well-meaning phrases that we've all heard, so many times.

> *I definitely feel I now have a voice. Belonging to a supportive community of women without children is not only empowering but at the same time normalising. I no longer feel so different and hence with the safety of our numbers I am brave.*
>
> Alizabeth: 41, Married, Australia

I watch them as they look around and begin to admire and identify with other women, feeling relieved to know that they are not alone in having been brought to their knees by childlessness. I hear their thinking start to shift as they begin to realise that maybe, just maybe, it's not all their own fault.

> *Meeting other women that understand my situation has been vital in my progress through grief. The friends I have met through Gateway Women have changed my life. My friend and I even flew from California to England for a Gateway Women retreat! The compassion that I got from these women was amazing! When you bare your soul to women that understand your heartache they become an instant sisterhood.*
>
> Kyla: 43, Married, USA

Then come the laughter and tears (often much more laughter than anyone was expecting!) as they work together to tease out hidden prejudices, to share their shame and watch it evaporate, to tentatively start forgiving themselves, their bodies, their choices, their fortunes and watch as new friendships form based on trust, respect and shared experience.

I was afraid that the women would be social misfits, which was completely untrue.

Sarah: 45, Single, USA

Women start arriving early and leaving late, meeting up with each other outside the group. They do their 'homework' assignments eagerly. They report breakthroughs. They start looking different, wearing different clothes and brighter colours. They report new and startling insights and conversations.

I was so excited to meet other childless women. Saying that, I was also apprehensive. Everyone's journey is so personal and taking that private pain outside of my comfort zone was definitely a challenge. It of course was so very worthwhile. I have met the most amazing women who are now very much part of my life.

Alizabeth: 41, Married, Australia

And then comes solidarity, sisterhood, a tribal bond. They come to understand that they're not alone, not freaks. Careers are reassessed, creative projects are taken up again, children in their life are embraced with affection not desperation, partners and parents are let off the hook. They start taking responsibility for their own happiness again.

They say it takes a whole village to raise a child. Well, I think it takes a whole tribe to heal a childless woman.

If you're feeling isolated in your childlessness, I can guarantee that there are other women nearby, almost definitely in your area, also sitting at home feeling marooned in a sea of mothers. You are not weird and you are not alone. You're part of at least one in five women. Find a way to connect with your tribe and it all starts to get a lot easier. Maybe even, dare I say it, *fun* again . . .

Elderhood Without Grandchildren

This is absolutely one of my biggest heartbreaks, watching the joy my mother experiences with her grandchildren and remembering the joyful times spent with my own grandmother. I don't think I will ever not wish to have had that experience; rather, life will be about creating other, different experiences.

Sally: 39, Married, Canada

Depending on how far along you are with your grief work, being around other people's grandchildren can be a joyful experience or a very challenging one. And sometimes, even if you're in a really good place about your childlessness, it can still be tiresome. (See more on working through 'Grandchildren Grief' in Chapter 4.) There are troubling issues for childless older men too, whom society increasingly finds suspect unless they have children, seeing them as potentially dangerous paedophiles.

I saw my brother carrying and entertaining his granddaughter recently and there was a pang of sadness about not experiencing that interaction and connection. It's a great shame, though, that wanting to be like that can be viewed as suspect if you don't have kids of your own, when often all we want to be is uncles or just caring men.

Robin: 55, In a Relationship, UK

Hopefully, by the time grandchildren come around, you'll have built a strong network of like-minded childless women who will act as a kind of inoculation against such feelings. I've found that having lots of childless women in my life who understand the delights and challenges of childlessness means that I am much more open and able to enjoy being around my friends with children, and listen to and empathise with their experience with interest and an open heart.

Stop Trying to Stay Young

Whatever age you are today, all of us are going to be childless older women in the future. And, as none of the current stereotypes for child-less older women is designed to make us feel good, this can make the idea of being comfortable in our skins as we age quite problematic! (See more on debunking childless stereotypes in Chapter 5.)

In some ways, the current cultural cult of unending youth and the fetishisation of motherhood are both ways of denying what comes after: the elder woman – what used to be called the 'crone'. The crone was as feared as she was revered – and yes, she could be a grumpy old woman as well as a wise and kindly old soul. Crones are human too, not fairy godmothers.

> I am happy in my life now and feel quite comfortable being a healthy sixty-four-year-old. I take pride in my grey hair and the many life lessons gleaned from 'an unexpected life'. I notice how a lot of women are very involved in the complexities and difficulties of the lives of their adult children and grandchildren; many feel trapped and burdened by the perceived demands and expectations of their families. I enjoy my off-the-mainstream life, the freedom to travel, to enjoy my work and to pursue many interests. And I acknowledge there are times when I would happily trade that freedom for a close relationship with a daughter and grandchildren, especially around Christmas and birthdays.
>
> Tilda: 64, Married, New Zealand

After all we've lived through and all we've endured and with mater-nal hearts that long to give to others, why *should* we go quietly into the night?

We have scars on our hearts but fire in our souls so why should we care if we don't look young anymore?

Hello! We're *not* young anymore and as soon as *we* stop having a problem with that or giving any headspace to the fact that others might have a problem with us still being here, things will get better for all women, mothers or not. And for older men too, who are beginning to experience increased ageism.[159]

> *I have been in denial about my age, perhaps linked to my shame at not having produced grandchildren. I've begun to lose the guilt, and enter this later stage of my life determined to experience joy and fun, and satisfaction in my work, all of the things that I have been denying myself for far too long.*
>
> Marianne: 63, Married, UK

If as intelligent, powerful older women we spend our time worrying about our looks, chasing after a vanished youth or lying about our age, we are, in effect, participating in our own shaming, our own invisibility. It is precisely *because* we don't have children (just as it was for many of the old healers and midwives) that we have the time to pursue knowledge for its own sake and to make shifts happen in our own lives and in our culture. How many of us have advanced degrees in more than one area, and are pursuing the love of learning for just that, love? How many of us train for second careers we are passionate about when we finally accept that we are never going to be mothers? How many of us have an enviable sparkle in our eyes that no cosmetic work can match because we've done the *internal* work to get our mojo working again?

What an asset we can be to the next generation if only we realise it and claim it. Hey, most people think we're invisible, so we can make all kinds of stuff happen before anyone's going to realise what we're up to!

The time has come to assert ourselves as powerful older women with opinions that matter. It's time to rebalance our society before it's too late and integrate the wisdom of the older women (both mothers *and* nomos) back into our world.

> *I'm now forty-four, single and I feel fantastic! I look forward to my elderhood as I've worked through many of the issues that were difficult in previous years. I recognise that a lot of my sadness about not having children was more about what I was going to do with my life, what was going to generate meaning and purpose for me, where I would feel a sense of family and belonging and what was going to be my life project. I recognise that a lot of my distress was caused by internalised shame – not being a parent, not having a partner ... that somehow I had failed to achieve these things in my life and therefore I was a failure. I now recognise that I haven't failed; in fact, quite the opposite.*

Eimear: 44, Single, Ireland

Only when masculine and feminine work hand in hand will we be able to create a fairer world for all. That's what feminism ultimately is about – equal rights, equal responsibility. We owe it to the generations that follow us, even if they're not our children, to leave things better than we found them.

We are the grown-ups – it's time we started acting like it and not running around worrying about our age, the size of our backside or what other people think of us.

Never before in recorded history have so many women like us been alive at the same time: intelligent, liberated, educated, financially independent women not involved in bringing up children. And never has the Western world seemed so in need of an injection of wise, compassionate, heartfelt thinking. If we childless women collectively realised our power, imagine how different things could be?

> *Childless women could play a big part in the revolution that we need. Ultimately, for an integrated solution to all these global problems we need all types of people, men/women, single/ married, parents/non-parents, all cultures, etc. Saying that, the Dalai Lama's quote about the world being saved by the Western woman is significant − more the 'woman' part rather than just Western ones, as women all over the world are changing the world in huge ways. There are in fact more female politicians and leaders in non-Western countries than in the West.*
>
> Selena: 50, Single, Australia/UK

Perhaps one of the single biggest fears that's holding us back from *claiming* that power is our fear of old age and what that might look like for us. In 2014 I was invited by Kirsty Woodard, a consultant and campaigner working in the ageing sector in the UK, to join her and two others to form AWOC, the Ageing Without Children collective,[160] and the attention from both individuals and the media has been huge. In the UK, at least 20 per cent of adults (men and women) currently in their forties will be ageing without children, yet it's still seen as a 'minority' issue.[161] That is the power of denial, both individually and collectively.

Old Lady Blues

Perhaps one of the most pernicious fears of childless women, particularly solo childless women, is not being sure who's going to take care of us when we're old and possibly frail. Even in our modern world, children are still seen as the answer to this fear.

> *I've come to realise that it's not that children are the answer to an adult's care needs when they're elderly, but that having children means that parents may not think through these difficult issues. As childless women, we don't have that luxury – we have to face the music now.*

Being old is a taboo in our society, obsessed as it is with youth, with control, with personal power and agency. The lack of obvious carers for elderly childless people brings every adult's unspoken fear out into the open. But rather than accept that this is an issue that everyone will face, a lot of the fear is projected back onto childless women with nasty 'joke' stereotypes like the 'crazy old cat lady'. Some research into this that I participated in, conducted by Dr Mary Pat Sullivan from Brunel University and Dr Mo Ray of Keele University in 2013, found that in fact the outcomes for single, childless elderly men are far more troubling.[162] Part of the remit of AWOC[163] is to make sure that both men's and women's needs are equally addressed.

> *I worry about having enough money for the nappy fund – there is very minimal state support where I live and my family genes predict ninety to ninety-five years ... and so I know that I must take steps now to be connected and in a community with others in similar positions so we can care for each other.*
>
> Velda: 45, Single, South Africa

Fears and Myths About Ageing Without Children

Myth 1: Having children guarantees that you will be taken care of when you're old

Research commissioned from IPSOS[164] by UK charity Stand Alone[165] in 2014 estimates that one in five families are affected by estrangement, and that five million people across the UK may be affected.[166] Of course, many

children (including ourselves) do indeed take care of their parents' needs
when old, but it's not a guarantee ...

- OK. First and most brutal question – how are you and your
  siblings (if you have any) getting on with your parents?

- Do you have plans to have your elderly parent(s) come and live
  with you when they need to? Do you have room for them physically and emotionally?

- Even if your relationship with your parents is very good, the
  reality is that it may be logistically impossible for you to give
  them a home in their old age. You may live on the other side of
  the country or world, or in a one-room flat that you're already
  stretched financially to afford.

- Also, who knows, you may die before your parents ...

- So, if you had had children, why would they too not have been
  subject to the same issues?

Myth 2: Having children guarantees grandchildren to keep you
company in your old age and bring some joy into your life
Although many grandparents do indeed enjoy the company of their grand-
children and find that they bring them joy, it's not a guarantee. Those of us
who will never have grandchildren need to be aware that the motherhood
myth creates a rose-tinted view of grandparenthood too.

- What if you'd had children and they didn't go on to have children,
  by choice or not? We of all people know that children are not a
  given!

- Your grandchildren might have ended up living on the other side
  of the world.

- You might not have liked your grandchildren very much or might
  have fallen out with their parents over the values they were
  bringing them up with.

- You might have found yourself having to be your grandchildren's
  primary carer whilst their parents worked full-time, and so what

you had hoped was going to be a bit of joy once a week turned into something which left you exhausted and resentful, [167] and perhaps also unable to get your teeth stuck into your 'third-age career', the one that might have topped up your retirement income.

• You might have enough joy in your own life by then, anyway! Who says only grandchildren can bring a sparkle to your eyes?! There's every chance that, with your Plan B (or Plan X, Y or Z) whizzing along, you'll be the one bringing joy into your own life and possibly into many others too!

• If you have children and young people in your life now who care about you (nephews, nieces, godchildren, young colleagues, mentees, friends' children), there's no reason to suppose that one or more of them might not be your ally in old age. They might even want to do it, rather than feel that they have to, because you're someone they love, cherish and admire and you've been a great mentor and role model to them of a life well lived.

Myth 3: You will be a helpless, senile old woman

AWOC, like Gateway Women, is desperately needed and could be a powerful voice, influencing many sectors, finding imaginative ways for people to age well and give back to society as well as being cared for.

Verity: 59, Divorced, UK

• Whilst old age does mean a decline in vitality, an unhealthy old age is not a given. A healthy lifestyle and an active mind *now* could make all the difference *then*. And a positive attitude and joyful heart can make it possible to have a happy old age even with unavoidable infirmities. We know, from our experience of childlessness, that the way we *think* about our situation is as important as the situation itself in how we cope with it. In fact, we're probably *better* equipped emotionally than many of our peers who have children to deal with the changes and challenges of old age.

- The Baby Boomer generation, currently just entering into old age, has changed everything it's passed through – relationships, education, work, love, parenting and spirituality. They're going to change 'old age' too. We're frightening ourselves with an old-fashioned idea of being elderly.

- Retirement is a phrase that will sound very quaint in generations to come; it's an unaffordable luxury for many and the changing demographics and life expectancy of our generation mean that quite a few of us will be on our third Plan B by the time we're of 'pensionable age'. Get your Plan B going now and you stand every chance of being a busy, connected and involved older woman. Our resourcefulness and knowledge acquired from navigating life without the identity of motherhood may become priceless as we move into old age.

- Care for the elderly is an issue that our generation needs to address before it's too late (well, it's already too late, but that's usually when things get done!). It needs to be sorted out for every-one because, even for those who *do* have children, those children cannot be relied upon to have the time, inclination or resources to advocate for and support their elderly parents when they need it. I believe that childless women, engaging in this issue in a proactive and helpful way, could have a big effect on changing not only the culture of ageing, but also the sense of childless women as some kind of 'burden' on society, or on future generations. Do take a look at the work AWOC[168] are doing and, if you're outside the UK, perhaps you could do something similar?

Myth 4: You will be a lonely old woman
Although loneliness is another social taboo, increasingly it is an aspect of modern life and in part can be attributed to the breakdown of extended family and community structures. Many parents also report feeling lonely.[169]

- Loneliness needs to be taken very seriously as it can have a gravely adverse effect on physical, emotional and mental health.[170] It's a fear that many adults have about their old age, but perhaps one that childless women (particularly those of us who are solo too) may fear more keenly. It's important to recognise that to counter this myth, you will need to take action to be 'part of' something. AWOC is developing groups around the UK and Gateway Women has free Meetup groups across the UK and Ireland, Europe, USA, Canada, Australia, New Zealand and Australia. There are also groups run by other organisations springing up around the world. The sooner you get involved with something that you can feel a part of, the better. (See Appendix for more details.)

- Some older women are great fun, appear to have a wide circle of inter-generational friends and are good at making contacts and friends in new situations. If that's what you're like as a person now, you'll hopefully still be like that as an old woman. And if not, there's still time to make changes, either internally or externally. Although I'm definitely less gregarious than I was in my twenties and thirties, I'm much more secure, and the warmth that used to be hidden under a brittle surface of bravado is now much more visible, which makes it easier for people to get to know me. I'm good at connecting with new people, good at keeping up with technology and I'm getting used to the fact that as a childless woman it's usually up to me to reach out and make new connections. Sometimes it gets a bit wearing, doing it all without the 'school gate club', but that's what organisations like Gateway Women are for – a new tribe, a different set of 'gates'.

- Loneliness is a part of life and it isn't to be feared if we have developed a good relationship with ourselves and with our 'source'. If we outlive our partner or don't have one and maybe outlive or are geographically distanced from our friends, there will probably be times of loneliness in later life. However, if we re-orient 'loneliness' as 'solitude' and welcome it as a time to go deeper within, we don't need to fear it. A fear of loneliness is, ultimately, a fear of ourselves. Isolation and boredom are different, and much harder to deal with. Hopefully we will have created such a rich life by then, full of meaning, that we won't have the time to be bored. I don't mean to downplay how crushing isolation feels – I've experienced it and would never belittle it, but it taught me a lot about myself and I faced and survived a really primal human fear.

- One of the best antidotes to loneliness I know is *giving*. As big-hearted women who longed to be mothers we have a lot to give and it's vital that we find a way to keep on giving as we grow older. Whether it's by being involved in our local community or the wider world, we can *always* find a way to contribute and we *must* do so in order to feel connected.

- As childless women we know what it is to live on the margins of society and we may already have suffered from being ostracised, isolated and lonely. Many of us have also experienced shame-based ideas about being 'wrong' or 'defective' and have not been able to avoid the sense of being alone in a vast universe by submerging ourselves into the identity of motherhood. As a result we're possibly *better* prepared for the falling away of famil-iar support, social structures, friends and family that so often accompanies advanced old age than most. We'll also be *better* prepared for some of the shocking ageism that's endemic in our cultures, having already dealt with sexism and pronatalism! We *know* that we need a strong network of like-minded, psycho-logically mature, emotionally generous and spiritually competent people to keep us sane and safe, and so we put time into building and sustaining those relationships. There is no reason to suppose that the skills it takes to make, honour and sustain networks will be any different in our old age. And, unlike our own grandparents, we will also be able to reach out and keep in touch via the internet and video-conferencing services. If you're someone who is resistant to computers, this might be the time to change your mind and book yourself onto a course whilst you're still young enough to become competent. You cannot afford your technophobia anymore – the price it may cost you later could be shockingly high.

Myth 5: You will die alone

- Anyone can die alone. It's a very human fear and to a great extent it's out of our control. I hope that my friends and family who have children do get to spend their last days together, but it can't be guaranteed. As our own parents age and we begin to have more experience with the complications of modern ageing and death we may begin to realise that it's really hard to *always* be there for a dying person, or to be sure to be with them at the moment of their death.

- Think about this: if you were to die in a month's time, would you die alone or would you die surrounded by friends and family wishing you well on your journey? In that case, why do you think that the person you're going to be when you are older is going to have such a different experience? When you think of yourself as an old woman, don't you realise that the person you're imagining isn't someone else – she's you! If you have friends and family who care for you now, do you think it's likely that you'll either fall out or lose touch with every single one of them by then, and that you won't make any new close connections? Don't you think that at least *one* of your nephews, nieces, godchildren, students, mentees, young colleagues or young friends might be around to sit with you, even if everyone else your own age has died? When you actually think about it, the fear of dying alone is a very human fear, and no more likely for us than for most people. Perhaps, because we're less sure who *might* be there with us, we may make a bit more preparation, and take better care of our friendships, just in case … Which can't be a bad thing, can it?

- We are in the wonderful position of being part of a generation that has a long expected lifespan. As Anne Karpf writes in her excellent short book *How to Age*, 'There has never been a better time to age.'[171] There are many ideas and experiments taking place around the world about how to create new types of living arrangements and communities. From the pioneering British Older Women's Co-housing Project[172] and the UK Co-housing Network[173] to innovative inter-generational schemes such as Shared Lives[174] and the situating of kindergartens in residential care facilities (to the delight and benefit of both groups),[175] there are many other ways to live out your elderhood than sitting at home alone, worrying about the bills ...

Thinking About Your Legacy

The idea of legacy was one that haunted me during my grieving, and I suspect it was one of the drivers behind some of my 'Mother Teresa' fantasies. It seemed terrifically important that I made a mark on this world; that I left something behind that showed I'd been here. I had no idea when I started my blog in 2011 that Gateway Women would evolve into what it has already become, and what I hope it has the potential to become. Hopefully it will be part of my 'legacy' but I can't say I think about it so much anymore; I'm much more concerned with the many, many things I'm excited about getting involved in before I die!

> I do not think of legacy. I think more of doing a good job now. However, if I can help create a saner, more loving world through my work I will feel good about my life.
>
> Margot: 67, Married, USA

What I have realised since coming out of my grief is that my life *already* had a legacy, I was just so consumed with what *hadn't* happened that I couldn't see it. Now I'm able to see myself and my life more evenly, I can accept that friends had often looked to me as a 'sensible head' in a crisis, and it turns out that one of them even says to herself, '*What would Jody do?*' when things get rocky! My nieces see me as a woman who has forged her own way in life and work despite several major setbacks, such as an industrial injury in my late twenties, the drama of being married to an alcoholic and my infertility. My mother sees me as someone who, like her, just keeps on getting up every time she's knocked down. Younger women see me as a mentor. Godchildren find me a calm port in a storm. Just recently, I was speaking with my oldest friend from schooldays (a mother of three) about legacy and she said, 'My life would have been poorer in so many ways without knowing you.' Legacy isn't always a 'thing'; often it's the trace we leave in the lives we touch, and sometimes we may never really know the impact we've had ...

Although I have inadvertently created a legacy with Gateway Women, I no longer feel I have something to make up for because I'm not a mother. The shame has gone. If you are spending a lot of time fretting about your legacy in this way, I hope that you too will find it eases as you become more comfortable with yourself.

For some of us, thinking about a legacy means thinking about to whom we are going to leave our money and possessions when we die. Having a will, and finding younger executors as well as friends or family our own age, is very important, and can feel quite challenging. AWOC is looking into exactly how to create a network of advocates that we can build trusting relationships with for later life if we don't have any young people it would be appropriate to ask.

I have no regrets about ageing without children myself, as I would loathe the thought that a child of mine would feel in any way obliged to look after me. I hope that my wide circle of friends will be generous and that the burden would be shared. I have prepared my will, power of lasting attorney and advance directive and I have chosen executors who are the daughters of a good friend of mine. They have been incredibly generous in agreeing to hold that responsibility if my good friends are unable to, if dead or too frail. I also know and trust the depth of empathy and integrity of these young women. I have also made provision that the executors are

there for major decisions only and that the detailed work would be
done by professionals.

Verity: 59, Divorced, UK

A life well lived is a precious thing, and the lessons learned in that
life deserve to be passed on. I often feel that having been denied the
opportunity to pass on our values, stories and wisdom to our children
or grandchildren is another invisible loss that we have to grieve. But
there are other ways that we can celebrate and pass on our wisdom.

I feel like I have already accomplished what I wanted to in terms
of leaving the world a better place through my work in recent
years. My next 'phase' will be a quiet, more private, subtler
journey, I believe, always keeping the earth and my caring for
her at the centre of my goals and decisions. Living lightly, leaving
little trace . . .

Sally: 39, Married, Canada

It might be that some of us, as we get older, find ways to contribute
to our community and to the following generations, although, as with
everything we do, *we'll* have to make it happen; there are no 'traditions'
for us to step into. Some examples of a legacy might be:

- A special relationship with a young person to whom you act as a
  mentor.

- A skill that you pass on.

- Your example as someone who has transformed pain into growth
  and came out of it with wisdom rather than bitterness.

- Your creative outputs: a book, a play, a painting, a garden, a
  business, an idea.

- A change in the way the younger generation in your extended
  family and community think about childlessness and their
  options.

* Your part in the wider 'nomo' movement.

* Your role in a cause or community.

We have a lot to offer; the world needs many caring, nurturing elders to turn the tide, given the environmental, social and economic challenges we face everywhere today.

Velda: 45, Single, South Africa

In the past, elders in society were valued as a source of wisdom. Indeed, in some Native American cultures it is believed that when a woman stops menstruating, her blood is retained inside her as wisdom instead. They also have a tradition that *all* elder women are known as 'grandmothers', whether mothers or not, and all are treated with respect and revered for their knowledge and wisdom. This continues in more traditional societies, such as some parts of the southern Mediterranean.

Can you imagine how much wisdom we'll have about how to create a life of meaning by the time we are old women? Does it seem sensible or acceptable that this knowledge is not passed on?

Before we get too carried away we need to remember that, in Western culture, ancestors are not revered down the generations. Indeed, how well do you know your own family history beyond that of your grandparents' generation? It is the fate of most of us to be forgotten by history, whether we have children or not. It is a normal and natural part of the cycle of life of which we are part. Yes, some individuals do leave their mark on history, but just because we're childless, we don't have to force ourselves to be one of them.

We Are the Role Models

If I had known that a happy and fulfilling life without children was possible, I might have begun the process of accepting my situation much earlier than I did. But when the alternative to motherhood looked so bleak that I couldn't even contemplate it, what choice did I have but to just keep on hoping, keep on planning, keep on dreaming and keep putting my life on hold in my quest to become a mother? Even just one role model of a woman I admired who was childless would have made a massive difference to me.

> *I am finding my voice and learning how to use it constructively; initially I was so ashamed and scared that I remained silent, but now I am speaking out. I am probably seen as a disturber of the peace – especially on Facebook! We are living in the information age and sharing our experience is so important, both so that others know that they are not alone, and to begin to shift societal thinking about those of us who are childless.*
>
> Velda: 45, Single, South Africa

For most of us, there are very few positive role models of childless women who spring immediately to mind and, of those that do, many of them will be childfree rather than childless as they are often more open about their situation. And as far as I'm aware from childfree women I've met, and from others whose books and articles I've read, they tend not to plumb the depths of grief over this decision the way that childless women do, although they are not free from it either as it's rarely the 'easy' decision that some imagine it to be.[176] And of course they're still subject to the same stigmas and exclusions as we are, plus the additional 'unnatural' tag, which is rarely, if ever, applied to a childfree man.

You may have noticed that when a woman in the public eye has children, she talks about them, even if it's to say that she *doesn't* talk about them. Yet, if she has no children and is past childbearing age, the topic is considered unmentionable. It's off limits, taboo unless it seems she's in politics, in which case it's often used against her, something which I wrote about in my *Guardian* article 'Julia Gillard and the fear of the childless woman'.[177] Unless an individual woman in the public eye chooses to talk about it, we are completely in the dark about her story – whether she's childfree or if she doesn't have children for one of the many complicated reasons that *we* all know so well. She's usually labelled with a stereotype (career woman, lesbian, unfeminine, etc.) and *her* side of the story is rarely heard or sought. The invisibility cloak goes on and that's that, it seems, case closed.

If childless women *do* get media attention, it's often to be pitied or as part of a news report about a woman in her fifties who's given birth, reinforcing the notion that we should 'never give up'. But what does that say about its alternative – coming to terms with childlessness? It says it's either not possible or that it has no value.

> *The most painful (and common) comments about my situation have been along the lines of 'you'll find someone' or 'there's still time' because they indicate that the listener finds the idea of ending up childless so abysmal that they can't even entertain it.*
>
> Sarah: 45, Single, USA

It seems that our current place is to be either a sob story or a miracle baby story, with not much in between. That's where we are today, but it will change – it's already changing and, with over 500 childless and childfree women role models in my Pinterest gallery, hopefully our experience will become increasingly normalised.[178]

As more and more of us seek the support to do our grief work and start working on our Plan B, the invisibility cloak will be dropped. As more and more of us put down the burden of shame society says is our lot, things will change.

*Just as we as individuals find change hard,
so does society. The change is happening, and
the media will reflect that, in time.*

Coming to terms with childlessness is hard, but it's worth it. After all, we've tried the alternative … It's vital, if future generations of women are not to suffer in silence, that we live our Plan B as unapologetically and frankly as possible.

> *It has been really hard to come to terms with my childlessness, and I have suffered a lot from shame and was afraid to tell my story. Once I started owning it and sharing it, it felt very freeing. One of the components of my own Plan B is that I'll be as open as possible to anyone who wants to know, so I'll be a trailblazer for women who are still getting to the other side of grief. I hope sharing my story will make it easier for them to be themselves and not feel left out, isolated or ashamed, like I used to. Yes, I've been called 'inspiring' and 'courageous' and other women have told me they look up to me. But all I do is try to live an authentic life. Being yourself shouldn't have to be inspiring and courageous. It should be easy, and I hope it will be in the near future.*
>
> Marjon: 43, Engaged, The Netherlands

*It is only by refusing to be ashamed that
the taboo of shame will be broken.*

Some of the things that need to come out in the open are:

- Talking about our childlessness and the impact it's had on our lives without shame or apology. We have a right to be sad. We have a right to our stories – including positive ones about creating a meaningful and fulfilling life without children. Each one is a piece of the mosaic of our times, our history.

- Getting the message out there that IVF is not a magic bullet and that more women and couples come out of fertility treatments *without* a family than the media coverage of miracle babies would suggest. The starker reality is that IVF is frontier science and in 2014 had a global failure rate of around 75 per cent.[179]

- Teenagers (both boys and girls) need to be taught about fertility as well as contraception to avoid the notion that getting pregnant later in life is 'easy'. Up to 30 per cent of fertility issues in couples are due to male-factor infertility; this is not a 'women's issue'.[180]

- To challenge the current thinking that makes the idea of having a family in your twenties and pursuing further education and a career later so unacceptable. If we're all going to live until we're almost a hundred and continue working in later life, what's the rush?

- To challenge the social and political structures that can make it so difficult for young professional women and couples to be able to combine careers and childrearing and thus have to leave it too late, or not be able to attempt it.

- It's time to get real about the issues between parents and non-parents within the workplace and look at how we can ensure that fairness, benefits and responsibilities go both ways.

- We need to speak up about the issues facing those ageing without children and get those *with* children to understand that if we can improve the prospects for people ageing without children, we will improve them for *everyone* (including, in time, *their* children).

- We need to finish the work that the sexual revolution began and make both men *and* women, both parents *and* non-parents, equally of value in our culture.

- It's time to challenge the 'business as usual'[181] model of pro-natalism and its insane over-privileging of parenting, which suggests that the answer to our problems as a society is always 'growth' (more children). Our planet is overpopulated and it's time we all faced up to the fact that, sadly, we need *fewer* children in the world right now, not more. We may not have chosen to be part of the solution by being childless, but it's possible that we are.

- To bridge the gap between mothers and non-mothers, between men and women, by showing that although our life experiences are different, our solidarity as *people* is more important. We need to shift our human consciousness from a 'role-based' one to a 'planetary'[182] one, and we need to do it *now*.

- There are many other things we need to speak out about too – how we are treated by our families, friends, employers, communities and our governments are just a few from a long list...

It is not necessary to be an activist in a stereotypical way; simply by living our lives openly and refusing to be shamed by our circumstances we are role models.

Childlessness is not the end of our story. It's the start of a new way of life – the life unexpected. There's no reason why our new lives can't be meaningful and fulfilling – and *whatever* that is will be unique to each of us.

Appendix

Gateway Women Resources

New resources are added regularly to this list on the Gateway Women website 'Resources' page. If you have any suggestions, do please get in touch: www.gateway-women.com. Links which start with 'bit.ly' are shortened versions of much longer links so that it's easier for you to type them into a search engine. They are case sensitive.

- **Gateway Women website (Global)**
  www.gateway-women.com
  Articles, courses, workshops, resources and blogs for childless women.

- **Gateway Women Private Online Community (Global)**
  www.gateway-women.com and click on 'Online Community'.
  All applications are vetted for member security and privacy.
  Free trial and either small membership fee or free thereafter.

- **Gateway Women Meetup Groups (UK and Ireland, Europe, USA, Canada, Australia, New Zealand, South Africa)**
  www.gateway-women.com and click on 'Find a Local Meetup'.
  Private social Meetup groups for childless women who wish to meet up in person.

- **Gateway Women Resource Library on Listly (Global)**
bit.ly/gw-library
An online library of articles and resources of relevance to childless women from global resources. At the last count almost 700 articles and resources.

- **Gateway Women Gallery of Childless and Childfree Role Models on Pinterest (Global)**
bit.ly/gw-role-models
Portraits and mini-biographies of childless and childfree women role models. 500+ women from different cultures and times, with more being added as I learn of them. Take a look and feel free to email me with your nominations.

Other Resources
(organised alphabetically by country)

CANADA

- **Femme Sans Enfant (French Canada)**
www.femmesansenfant.com
Blogs, articles and video interviews with childless and childfree women (and men) across the Francophone world. Started by Catherine-Emmanuelle Delisle, who is childless due to early menopause (age fourteen). It won in the 2014 'Activism and Social Justice' category in Canada's 'Schmutzie' Weblog Awards. Also a Meetup group: www.meetup.com/femme-sans-enfant

- **Mothering Your Heart (English-speaking Canada/Global)**
www.motheringyourheart.com
Email programme and group for support after infertility and baby loss.

FRANCE

● **Not About Kids**
www.notaboutkids.com
A social and campaigning group for men and women without
children by choice or not. Also a Meetup group.

IRELAND

● **Childfree in Ireland**
www.childfreeinireland.wordpress.com
A blog and list of resources for people without children living in
Ireland.

SWEDEN

● **Andra sidan tröskeln**
www.andrasidantroskeln.se
A blog for involuntarily childless women in Sweden. Also a
Facebook and Meetup group.

THE NETHERLANDS

● **Eigen Plan Coaching**
www.eigenplan.nl
Marjon Bakker's website, blog and coaching programme for Dutch
women coming to terms with involuntary childlessness.

NEW ZEALAND

● **Teresa Woodham**
www.teresawoodham.com
A childless psychotherapist, Teresa offers workshops and individual sessions for involuntarily childless women.

UNITED KINGDOM

- **BICA (British Infertility Counselling Association)**
www.bica.net
The BICA website has a list of registered infertility counsellors in the UK. It is an organisation that is very aware of the support that men, women and couples need to move on with their lives after childlessness. It has been very supportive of the work of Gateway Women.

- **Campaign to End Loneliness**
www.campaigntoendloneliness.org/about-loneliness
This is both a campaigning group and also provides support. Lots of ways you can get involved, whatever your age or situation.

- **Childless Stepmothers**
www.childlessstepmums.co.uk
This UK-based internet forum describes itself as 'a sanctuary for women thrown into an instant family of often angry ex-wives, resentful stepchildren and guilty or mourning fathers'.

- **The Daisy Network**
www.daisynetwork.org.uk
A UK charity that supports women who have experienced premature menopause or 'premature ovarian failure', as it's often referred to.

- **The Dovecote**
www.thedovecote.org
A UK website and organisation for women who are involuntarily childless. Also an online community and workshops.

- **Give Sorrow Words**
www.gilltunstallcounselling.co.uk
London-based counsellor Gill Tunstall runs regular 'Give Sorrow Words' ceremonies. These are non-denominational memorial

ceremonies for anyone who has experienced losses associated with fertility or unwanted childlessness.

- **More to Life**
www.infertilitynetworkuk.com/more_to_life
A UK charity that provides online and face-to-face groups for women and couples moving on after infertility treatment.

- **Saying Goodbye**
www.sayinggoodbye.org
Saying Goodbye organise non-denominational services of remembrance in cathedrals across the UK. The services are for people who have lost a child at any age or stage of pregnancy, at birth or in infancy, whether it was recently or many years ago.

- **Wanted to be a Dad**
www.wantedtobeadad.com
British Academic and childless man Robin Hadley's website for involuntarily childless men.

USA

- **Bella de Paulo's 'Community of Single People'**
bit.ly/single-community
This is a closed Facebook group for 'Single people who want to live single lives joyfully, and free of stereotyping and stigma'. This group is for all genders, and includes single parents. It has nothing to do with dating. Bella de Paulo is an academic and writer who writes on the prejudices experienced by single adults, and coined the term 'matrimania'.

- **Childless by Marriage**
www.childlessbymarriageblog.com
Writer and musician Sue Fagalde Lick's book and blog about life as a childless stepmother and now as a childless widow.

- **Childless Mothers Connect (CMC) and Childless Mothers Adopt (CMomA)**
  www.cmoma.org/cmc
  Psychotherapist Dr Marcy Cole's website, organisation and community for 'Childless Mothers' (by both choice and circumstance) and her project (CMomA) to connect children-in-need with adoptive or foster mothers. Marcy is a childless woman herself.

- **Life Without Baby**
  www.lifewithoutbaby.com
  Lisa Manterfield's blog, online community, online courses and resources for women coming to terms with life as a childless woman. Lisa is the author of *I'm Taking my Eggs and Going Home*.

- **The Mother Within**
  www.themotherwithin.com
  Events, equine healing retreats and Facebook community for involuntarily childless women created by Christine Erickson, author of *The Mother Within*.

- **Our Spirit Babies**
  www.spiritbabies.org
  Interfaith community events for people who have been affected by pregnancy loss, whether by miscarriage, abortion, stillbirth or for any other reason. Those mourning not being able to have children for any reason are also welcome.

- **Resolve**
  www.resolve.org
  The US National Infertility Association with many local groups and a fantastic website.

- **Savvy Auntie**
  www.savvyauntie.com
  Melanie Notkin's organisation and online community for women

without children who are aunts, godmothers or in some way 'childful'. She also writes movingly for Huffington Post on being a single, childless woman in her mid-forties. www.huffingtonpost.com/melanie-notkin

Recommended Reading

As there are more and more books being published that are relevant to us, this list keeps growing, I'm happy to say! Check out www.gateway-women.com 'Resources' to read my mini-reviews of each one, and to see the latest additions.

All the books listed below can also be found online at bit.ly/LTLU-Bluebird.

On social and cultural aspects of childlessness

- Cannold, L. (2005) *What, No Baby? Why women are losing the freedom to mother and how they can get it back.* Freemantle, Australia: Curtin University Books.
  bit.ly/what-no-baby
  www.cannold.com

- Carroll, L. (2012) *The Baby Matrix: Why Freeing Our Minds from Outmoded Thinking About Parenting and Reproduction Will Create a Better World.* USA: Live True Books.
  bit.ly/baby-matrix
  www.lauracarroll.com

- Erikson, C. (2015) *The Mother Within: A Guide To Accepting Your Childless Journey.* USA/Global Kindle e-book.
  bit.ly/mother within
  www.themotherwithin.com

- Holmes, M. (2014). *The Female Assumption: A Mother's Story, Freeing Women from the View that Motherhood is a Mandate.* USA: CreateSpace.
  bit.ly/female-assumption
  www.melanieholmesauthor.com

On the solo childless experience

- Cagen, S. (2004) *Quirky Alone: A Manifesto for Uncompromising Romantics.* USA, New York: HarperSanFrancisco, HarperCollins Publishers.
  bit.ly/quirky-alone
  www.quirkyalone.net/

- DePaulo, B. (2007) *Singled Out: How Singles Are Stereotyped, Stigmatized, and Ignored, and Still Live Happily Ever After.* USA, New York: St Martin's Press.
  bit.ly/singled-out
  www.belladepaulo.com
  bit.ly/single-community

- Eckel, S. (2014) *It's Not You: 27 (Wrong) Reasons You're Single.* USA, New York: Perigree (Penguin Group).
  bit.ly/eckel-single
  www.saraeckel.com

- Feldon, B. (2003) *Living Alone and Loving It: A Guide to Relishing the Solo Life.* USA, New York: Simon & Schuster.
  bit.ly/living-alone

- Notkin, M. (2014) *Otherhood: Modern Women Finding a New Kind of Happiness.* USA, New York: Seal Press.
  bit.ly/otherhood
  www.huffingtonpost.com/melanie-notkin
  www.savvyauntie.com

On midlife and growing older without children

- Athill, D. (2009) *Somewhere Towards the End.* UK: Granta Books.
  bit.ly/athill-towards-end
  www.grantabooks.com/Diana-Athill

- Bolen, J. S. (2001) *Goddesses in Older Women: Archetypes for Women Over Fifty.* USA, New York: HarperCollins.
  bit.ly/bolen-goddess

- Gross, J. (2011) *A Bittersweet Season: Caring for our Aging Parents – and Ourselves.* USA, New York: Random House Publishing Group.
  bit.ly/janegross
  www.newoldage.blogs.nytimes.com

- Karpf, A. (2014) *How to Age.* UK, London: The School of Life, Pan Macmillan.
  bit.ly/howtoage

- Northrup, C. (2015) *Goddesses Never Age: The Secret Prescription for Radiance, Vitality and Wellbeing.* UK/USA: Hay House.
  bit.ly/northrup-goddess
  www.drnorthrup.com

- Robertson, G. (2014) *How to Age Positively: A Handbook of Personal Change for Later Life.* UK, Bristol: Positive Ageing Associates.
  bit.ly/age-positively

- Williamson, M. (2008) *The Age of Miracles: Embracing the New Midlife.* UK: Hay House.
  bit.ly/marianne-miracles
  www.marianne.com

On doing your grief work

* Beattie, M. (1990) *The Language of Letting Go.* USA, Minnesota: Hazelden Publishing.
  bit.ly/melanie-letting-go
  www.melodybeattie.net

* Beattie, M. (2006) *The Grief Club: The Secret for Getting Through All Kinds of Change.* USA, Minnesota: Hazelden Publishing.
  bit.ly/grief-club
  www.melodybeattie.net

* Biziou, B. (2006) *The Joy of Ritual: Spiritual Recipes to Celebrate Milestones, Ease Transitions, and Make Every Day Sacred.* USA: Cosimo Books.
  bit.ly/childless-ritual
  www.barbarabiziou.com

* Chodron, P. (1997) *When Things Fall Apart: Heart Advice for Difficult Times.* UK, London: Element / HarperCollins
  bit.ly/chodron
  www.pemachodronfoundation.org

* Cleantis, T. (2015). *The Next Happy: Let Go of the Life You Planned and Find a New Way Forward.* USA, Minnesota: Hazelden Publishing.
  bit.ly/nexthappy
  www.traceycleantis.com

* Kübler-Ross, E. and Kessler, D. (2005) *On Grief and Grieving: Finding the Meaning of Grief Through the Five Stages of Loss.* UK, London: Simon & Schuster.
  bit.ly/grief-and-grieving
  www.ekrfoundation.org

- Manterfield, L. (2014) *Workbook 1: Letting Go of the Dream of Motherhood* (Life Without Baby Workbook Series) Amazon Kindle. www.lifewithoutbaby.com/books

On understanding and embracing your Inner Bitch

- Ahlers, A. and Arylo, C. (2015) *Reform Your Inner Mean Girl: 7 Steps to Stop Bullying Yourself and Start Loving Yourself.* USA, New York: Atria Books / Simon & Schuster.
  bit.ly/inner-mean-girl
  www.innermeangirlreformschool.com

- Brown, B. (2010) *The Gifts of Imperfection: Let Go of Who You Think You're Supposed to Be and Embrace Who You Are.* USA, Minnesota: Hazelden Publishing.
  bit.ly/brene-gifts
  www.brenebrown.com

- Cantopher, C. (2003) *Depressive Illness: The Curse of the Strong.* UK, London: Sheldon Press.
  bit.ly/cantopher
  bit.ly/cantopher-pdf [Short overview]

- Ford, D. (2001) *Dark Side of the Light Chasers: Reclaiming Your Power, Creativity, Brilliance and Dreams.* London, UK: Hodder.
  bit.ly/ford-dark
  www.debbieford.com

- Goldstein, E. (2015). *Uncovering Happiness: Overcoming Depression Through Mindfulness and Self-Compassion.* UK, London: Simon & Schuster.
  bit.ly/uncovering-happiness
  www.elishagoldstein.com

- Neff, K. (2011) *Self-Compassion: Stop Beating Yourself Up and Leave Insecurity Behind.* UK: Hodder and Stoughton.
  bit.ly/neff-compassion
  www.self-compassion.org

On forgiving your body

- Brown, B. (2007) *I Thought It Was Just Me: Making the Journey from 'What Will People Think?' to 'I Am Enough'.* USA: Gotham Books.
  bit.ly/brene-shame
  www.brenebrown.com

- Brown, B. (2012) *Listening to Shame* [Online Video].
  bit.ly/brene-ted-shame
  www.brenebrown.com

- Roth, G. (2011) *Women, Food & God: An Unexpected Path to Almost Everything.* UK: Simon & Schuster.
  bit.ly/roth-food
  www.geneenroth.com

- Wolf, N. (1998) *The Beauty Myth: How Images of Beauty are Used Against Women.* UK: Vintage Books.
  bit.ly/beauty-myth
  www.naomiwolf.org

- Zackheim, V. (2007) Ed. *For Keeps: Women Tell the Truth About Their Bodies, Growing Older, and Acceptance.* UK: Avalon Publishing Group.
  bit.ly/for-keeps
  www.victoriazackheim.com

On meaning, purpose, happiness and choices

- Beck, M. (2001) *Finding Your Own North Star: How to Claim the Life You Were Meant to Live.* UK, London: Piatkus Books.
  bit.ly/beck-north-star
  www.marthabeck.com

- Frankl, V. E. (1946) *Man's Search for Meaning.* UK, London: Ebury Publishing.
  bit.ly/frankl-meaning-1946

- Frankl, V. E. (1947) *Man's Search for Ultimate Meaning.* With a Foreword by Claudia Hammond (2011) UK, London: Rider, Ebury Publishing.
  bit.ly/frankl-ultimate

- Hollis, J. (2005) *Finding Meaning in the Second Half of Life: How to Finally, Really, Grow Up.* USA, New York: Gotham / Penguin Books.
  bit.ly/hollis-meaning

- Ricard, M. (2006) *Happiness: A Guide to Developing Life's Most Important Skill.* UK, London: Atlantic Books.
  bit.ly/ricard-happiness
  www.en.wikipedia.org/wiki/Matthieu_Ricard

- Salecl, R. (2010) *Choice.* UK, London: Profile Books.
  bit.ly/salecl-choice
  An animated version of Renata Salecl lecturing on 'Choice'
  bit.ly/salecl-rsa-choice

- Ditzler, J. (1994) *Your Best Year Yet: The 10 Questions that will change your life forever.* UK, London: Harper Element.
  bit.ly/ditzler-best-year-yet

- Dickson, M. (2010) *Please Take One: One Step Towards a More Generous Life.* UK, London: The Generous Press.
  www.pleasetakeonestep.com

On developing your creativity (and dealing with your resistance)

- Cameron, J. (1995) *The Artist's Way: A Course in Discovering and Recovering Your Creative Self.* UK, London: Pan Books.
  bit.ly/cameron-artist
  www.juliacameronlive.com

- Lamott, A. (2008) *Bird by Bird: Some Instructions on Writing and Life.* USA: Scribe Publications.
  bit.ly/lamott-bird
  www.facebook.com/AnneLamott

- MacLeod, H. (2009). *Ignore everybody: and 39 other keys to creativity.* USA, New York: Portfolio (Penguin Books).
  bit.ly/hugh-creativity
  www.gapingvoid.com

- McNiff, S. (1998) *Trust the Process: An Artist's Guide to Letting Go.* USA: Shambala Publications.
  bit.ly/mcniff-process

- Pressfield, S. (2003) *The War of Art: Break Through the Blocks and Win Your Inner Creative Battles.* UK: Orion.
  bit.ly/pressfield-war
  www.blackirishbooks.com

On connecting and reconnecting to source and self-care

- Ban Breathnach, S. (2003). *Romancing the Ordinary: A Year of Everyday Indulgences.* USA, New York: Simon & Schuster.
  bit.ly/romancing-the-ordinary

- Beck, M. (2011). *Finding Your Way in a Wild New World: Reclaim Your True Nature to Create the Life You Want.* USA, New York: Simon & Schuster.
  bit.ly/kempton-meditation
  www.sallykempton.com

* Kempton, S. (2011) *Meditation for the Love of It: enjoying your own deepest experience.* Forward by Elizabeth Gilbert. USA, Boulder, Colorado: Sounds True Inc.
  bit.ly/wordlessness
  www.marthabeck.com

* Macy, J. and Johnstone, C. (2012) *Active Hope: How to Face the Mess We're In Without Going Crazy.* USA, Novato, CA: New World Library.
  bit.ly/active-hope
  www.joannamacy.net

* Plotkin, B. (2003) *Soulcraft: crossing into the mysteries of nature and psyche.* USA, Novato, CA: New World Library.
  bit.ly/soul-craft-plotkin
  www.animas.org

* Prendergast, J. J. (2015) *In Touch: How to Tune Into the Inner Guidance of Your Body and Trust Yourself.* USA, Boulder, Colorado: Sounds True Inc.
  bit.ly/prendergast-in-touch
  www.listeningfromsilence.com

On thinking about changing your work/career as part of your Plan B

* Krznaric, R. (2012) *How to Find Fulfilling Work.* The School of Life. UK, London: Macmillan.
  bit.ly/roman-work
  www.romankrznaric.com

* Williams, J. (2010) *Screw Work, Let's Play: How to Do What You Love and Get Paid for It.* UK, London: Pearson Business.
  bit.ly/williams-work
  www.screwworkletsplay.com

- Williams, N. (1999) *The Work We Were Born to Do: Find the Work You Love, Love the Work You Do.* UK, Kent: Balloon View Publishing.
  bit.ly/born-to-do
  www.iamnickwilliams.com

Other women's stories

- Black, R. and Scull, L. (2005) *Beyond Childlessness: For Every Woman Who Wanted To Have a Child – and Didn't.* UK: Rodale Books.
  bit.ly/beyond-childlessness
  www.beyondchildlessness.com

- Carter, J. W. and Carter, M. (1998) *Sweet Grapes: How to Stop Being Infertile and Start Living Again.* USA: Perspectives.
  bit.ly/sweet-grapes

- Comstock, K. and Comstock, B. (2013) *Honouring Missed Motherhood: Loss, Choice & Creativity.* USA, Ashland, Oregon: Willow Press.
  bit.ly/missed-motherhood
  www.missedmotherhood.com

- Daum, M. (2015). *Selfish, Shallow and Self-Absorbed: Sixteen Writers on the Decision NOT to have Kids.* Edited and with an Introduction by Meghan Daum. USA, New York: Picador (Macmillan).
  bit.ly/daum-selfish
  www.meghandaum.com

- De Ridder, N. and Nick W. (2013) *Just The Two of Us: Giving New Meaning to Our Lives Through Dealing with Infertility.* UK: Epubli.
  bit.ly/ridder-two-of-us

- Fagalde Lick, S. (2012) *Childless by Marriage* US: Blue Hydrangea Productions.
www.childlessbymarriageblog.com

- Brooks Froelker, J. (2015) *Ever Upward: Overcoming the Lifelong Losses of Infertility to Own a Childfree Life.* USA: Morgan James.
bit.ly/ever-upward
www.everupward.org

- Hepburn, J. (2014) *The Pursuit of Motherhood. UK: Troubadour Publishing.*
bit.ly/jessica-pursuit
www.thepursuitofmotherhood.com

- Manterfield, L. (2010) *I'm Taking My Eggs and Going Home: How One Woman Dared to Say No to Motherhood.* USA: Steel Rose Press.
bit.ly/eggs-home
www.lifewithoutbaby.com

- Mahoney Tsingdinos, P. (2010) *Silent Sorority: A (Barren) Woman Gets Busy, Angry, Lost and Found.* USA: Booksurge Plc.
bit.ly/silent-sorority
www.silentsorority.com

- Walker, E. L. (2011) *Complete Without Kids: An Insider's Guide to Childfree Living by Choice or by Chance.* USA, Austin: Greenleaf Book Group Press.
bit.ly/complete-without-kids
www.completewithoutkids.com

- Yvette, P., Ann, R., and Lynne, J. (2012) *Being Fruitful Without Multiplying: Stories and Essays from Around the World.* USA, Seattle: Coffeetown Enterprises.
bit.ly/without-multiplying
www.coffeetownpress.com

Acknowledgements

Thank you to Katie James at Macmillan and Carole Tonkinson, Olivia Morris and Anna Bowen at Bluebird for your enthusiasm and guidance every step of the way for this new edition of my book.

A huge and heartfelt thank you to the childless women and men who generously shared their stories. All names have been changed where requested, but they and I know who they are. Some of you had to return to some of the darkest times in your lives to share your experiences, and I know that wasn't easy. It's wonderful to have your voices as part of this book and I hope they will help many more people than just my voice alone. Thank you so very much.

Thank you also to: Elly and Mark, for their belief, support and love.

Diane Osgood, for seeing the potential in GW from so early on, and for lending me her mountain hideaway to create this new edition.

'Team Jody': Helen Burke, Natalie Kontarsky, Sarah Hudson, Liz Sutton, Emily Parikh, Lucy Firmin, Maggie Rogers, Kris Black, Tai Long and ZZ.

The teaching staff and my fellow students at Terapia Institute including Bozena Merrick, Lucy Templeton, Jonathan Harris, Lizzie Smosarski, Clare Soloway, Di Gammage, Alex Noble and Andrea Katz.

Christian, Sophy, Tom, Jane and all the deF's and Newts for being the best outlaw family a divorcee could wish for.

My supportive and understanding friends who've put up with hardly seeing me because I've either been working, writing or studying for the last few years: Alexis Walters, Anna Kendall, Chloe Cunningham, Diane Metta, Janet Murray, Jo Wyeth, Marie Valensi, Mark Luscombe-Whyte, Neil Stott, Nell Willis, Nunzio Lanotte, Sam Hunter, Sophie Lem, Stella Michael, Valerie James.

And last but never least, to all the courageous, vulnerable, funny, inspiring, creative, generous and loving childless women I have had the honour and delight to have met and worked with since I started writing my blog in 2011. I've come a long way from feeling like the only childless woman in the world thanks to you. You're one heck of a tribe!

Endnotes

All these endnotes are also accessible online as a Listly list – bit.ly/LTLU-Bluebird (case sensitive).

1 Keizer, R. (2010) 'Remaining childless: Causes and consequences from a life course perspective': Dissertation: Utrecht University. Data is not within dissertation as it is an estimate only, and based on data drawn from the Netherlands and the United States, but is referred to here in an article about Professor Keizer's research. www.nwo.nl/actueel/nieuws/2010/Kinderloosheid+is+zelden+een+keuze.html (Accessed: October 2015).

2 Lehrer, J. (2007) *Proust Was a Neuroscientist.* New York: Houghton Mifflin Harcourt.

3 Office for National Statistics (UK) *Cohort Fertility 2010* (online). www.ons.gov.uk/ons/rel/fertility-analysis/cohort-fertility--england-and-wales/2010/cohort-fertility-2010.html (Accessed: August 2015).

4 Frejka, T. (2008) 'Completed family size in Europe: Incipient decline of the two-child family model?' Demographic Research, Volume (19) pp.47–72. www.demographic-research.org/volumes/vol19/4/19-4.pdf (Accessed: August 2015).

5 Nicolson, V. (2007) *Singled Out: How Two Million Women Survived Without Men after the First World War.* UK: Viking.

6 It is challenging to find comparable statistics from around the world, as different countries and organisations collect the data differently, and

censuses/surveys do not always cover the same periods. For example, for many countries, the data they report is childlessness in women aged 40–44, which therefore doesn't take into account the many births that now happen in that period, either naturally or with the help of fertility treatments. The UK collects childlessness data on women aged 45 (the last day before their 46th birthday), which possibly reflects a more accurate figure.

7 United Nations, Department of Economic and Social Affairs: Population Division. 'World Fertility Report 2013: Fertility at the Extremes' (online), United Nations: New York, 2014. www.un.org/en/development/desa/population/publications/fertility/world-fertility-2013.shtml (Accessed: August 2015).

8 Office for National Statistics, UK (2014). Statistical bulletin: 'Childbearing for Women Born in Different Years, England and Wales, 2013'. www.ons.gov.uk/ons/rel/fertility-analysis/childbearing-for-women-born-in-different-years/2013/stb-cohort-fertility-2013.html#tab-Childlessness. (Accessed: August 2015).

9 OECD (2014) SF2.5: Childlessness. OECD – Social Policy Division – Directorate of Employment, Labour and Social Affairs (online). www.oecd.org/els/family/database.htm (Accessed: October 2015).

10 Pew Research Centre, USA (2015). 'Childlessness Falls, Family Size Grows Amongst Highly Educated Women' (online). www.pewsocialtrends.org/2015/05/07/childlessness-falls-family-size-grows-among-highly-educated-women/ (Accessed: August 2015).

11 PewResearch Centre, USA (2010) 'Childlessness' (online). www.pewsocialtrends.org/2015/05/07/childlessness/ (Accessed August 2015).

12 Astone, N. M., Martin, S. and Peters, H. E. (2015) 'Millennial Childbearing and the Recession' Urban Institute, Washington DC, USA. www.urban.org/research/publication/millennial-childbearing-and-recession (Accessed: August 2015).

13 United Nations, Department of Economic and Social Affairs, Population Division. 'World Fertility Report 2013: Fertility at the Extremes' (online). United Nations: New York, 2014. www.un.org/en/development/desa/population/publications/fertility/world-fertility-2013.shtml (Accessed: August 2015).

14 Government of Canada: Statistics Canada. 2011 Census (online). www12.statcan.gc.ca/census-recensement/index-eng.cfm (Accessed: October 2015).

15 Renzetti, E. (2013) 'Why childless people are persecuted' (online). *Globe and Mail* (Canada): Wednesday 18 May 2013. www.theglobeandmail. com/life/parenting/why-childless-people-are-persecuted/ article12005541/?page=all (Accessed: August 2015).

16 O'Connor, J. (2012) 'Trend of couples not having children just plain selfish' (online). *National Post* (Canada): 19 September 2012. www.news. nationalpost.com/full-comment/joe-oconnor-selfishness-behind-growing-trend-for-couples-to-not-have-children (Accessed: August 2015).

17 Australian Bureau of Statistics (2012) 412.0 'Australian Social Trends', 2002. www.abs.gov.au/AUSSTATS/abs@.nsf/ bb8db737e2af84b8ca2571780015701e/1e8c8e4887c33955ca2570ec000a 9fe5!OpenDocument (Accessed: August 2015).

18 Statistics New Zealand (2012) 'More Women Are Remaining Childless' (online). www.stats.govt.nz/browse_for_stats/population/mythbusters/ more-women-remain-childless.aspx (Accessed August 2015).

19 Chemin, A. (2015). 'France's baby boom secret: get women into work and ditch rigid family norms', *Guardian*, Saturday 21 March 2015. www.theguardian.com/world/2015/mar/21/france-population-europe-fertility-rate (Accessed: August 2015).

20 Kramer, S. P. (2014) 'Sweden Pushed Gender Equality to Boost Birth Rates', We-News, 27 April 2014. www.womensenews.org/story/the-world/140426/sweden-pushed-gender-equality-boost-birth-rates (Accessed: August 2015).

21 Mesco, M. (2014) 'More Italian Women Are Choosing to Have No Children', *Wall Street Journal*, 22 April 2014. www.graphics.wsj.com/ italys-women-shun-childbearing/ (Accessed: August 2015).

22 Hara, T. (2008). 'Increasing Childlessness in Germany and Japan: Toward a Childless Society?' International Journal of Japanese Sociology, 2008, Number 17. Blackwell Publishing Ltd (online). www.onlinelibrary. wiley.com/doi/10.1111/j.1475-6781.2008.00110.x/full (Accessed: August 2015).

23 Mesco, M. (2014) 'More Italian Women Are Choosing to Have No

Children', *Wall Street Journal*, 22 April 2014. www.graphics.wsj.com/ italys-women-shun-childbearing/ (Accessed: August 2015).

24 United Nations, Department of Economic and Social Affairs: Population Division. 'World Fertility Report 2013: Fertility at the Extremes' (online). United Nations: New York, 2014. www.un.org/en/development/desa/ population/publications/fertility/world-fertility-2013.shtml Page 64. (Accessed: August 2015).

25 Miettinen, A., Rotkirch, A., Ivett Szalma, I., Donno, A. and Tanturri, M. (2014). 'Increasing childlessness in Europe: time trends and country differences', Väestöliiton Väestöntutkimuslaitoksen työpaperi (The Population Research Institute) 2014 (5). Working paper no 5. www.familiesandsocieties.eu (Accessed: August 2015).

26 Hara, T. (2008). 'Increasing Childlessness in Germany and Japan: Toward a Childless Society?' *International Journal of Japanese Sociology*, 2008, Number 17. Blackwell Publishing Ltd (online). www.onlinelibrary.wiley. com/doi/10.1111/j.1475-6781.2008.00110.x/full (Accessed: August 2015).

27 United Nations, Department of Economic and Social Affairs: Population Division. 'World Fertility Report 2013: Fertility at the Extremes' (online). United Nations: New York, 2014. www.un.org/en/development/desa/ population/publications/fertility/world-fertility-2013.shtml Page 13. (Accessed: August 2015).

28 United Nations, Department of Economic and Social Affairs: Population Division. 'World Fertility Report 2013: Fertility at the Extremes' (online). United Nations: New York, 2014. www.un.org/en/development/desa/ population/publications/fertility/world-fertility-2013.shtml Page 3. (Accessed: August 2015).

29 Wikipedia (2013) 'Combined oral contraceptive pill' (online). Available at: www.en.wikipedia.org/wiki/Combined_oral_contraceptive_pill (Accessed October 2015).

30 *Science Daily* (2012) 'Late Motherhood: A Selfish Choice?' (online). Available at: www.sciencedaily.com/releases/2012/09/120903143056. htm (Accessed October 2015).

31 Bennett, J. (2015) 'A Masters Degree in ... Masculinity?' *New York Times* (online). 8 August, 2015. www.nytimes.com/2015/08/09/ fashion/masculinities-studies-stonybrook-michael-kimmel.html (Accessed: October 2015).

32 Hanisch, C. (1969) 'The Personal Is Political, Notes from the Second Year: Women's Liberation' (1970) ed. Koedt, A. and Firestone, S. (online). Available at: www.carolhanisch.org/CHwritings/PIP.html (Accessed October 2015).

33 ESHRE – European Society of Human Reproduction and Embryology (online). ART Fact Sheet (July 2014). www.eshre.eu/Guidelines-and-Legal/ART-fact-sheet.aspx (Accessed: October 2015).

34 Cannold, L. (2005) *What, No Baby? Why women are losing the freedom to mother and how they can get it back.* Australia, Freemantle: Curtin University Books.

35 Orange, R. (2012) 'All dads together: my new life among Sweden's latte pappas', *Observer*. Sunday 18 November 2012. www.guardian.co.uk/money/2012/nov/18/swedish-latte-pappa-shared-childcare?INTCMP=SRCH (Accessed: October 2015).

36 Speech by Prime Minister Stefan Löfven at the Third International Conference on 'Financing for Development: 'Financing for gender equality – results and good practices'. 15 July 2015. (online). www.government.se/speeches/2015/07/financing-for-gender-equality--results-and-good-practices/ (Accessed: August 2015).

37 Chemin, A. (2015). 'France's baby boom secret: get women into work and ditch rigid family norms', *Guardian*, Saturday 21 March 2015. www.theguardian.com/world/2015/mar/21/france-population-europe-fertility-rate (Accessed: August 2015).

38 Alcorn, K. and Moses, L. (2011) '10 Reasons It's Easier to Be a Working Mom in France' (online). USA: Working Moms Break. January 26, 2011. www.workingmomsbreak.com/2011/01/26/10-reasons-its-easier-to-be-a-working-mom-in-france/ (Accessed: August 2015).

39 Chemin, A. (2015). 'France's baby boom secret: get women into work and ditch rigid family norms', *Guardian*, Saturday 21 March 2015. www.theguardian.com/world/2015/mar/21/france-population-europe-fertility-rate (Accessed: August 2015).

40 Doughty, S. (2015) 'Working mothers risk damaging their child's prospects', *Mail Online* (online). Tuesday 11 August, 2015. www.dailymail.co.uk/news/article-30342/Working-mothers-risk-damaging-childs-prospects.html (Accessed: August 2015).

41 Niles, E. (2015). 'New Report Shows the Powerful Effect of Working

Moms', *Ms Magazine* (online). 17 July 2015. www.msmagazine.com/blog/2015/07/17/new-report-shows-the-powerful-effect-of-working-moms/ (Accessed: August 2015).

42 European Union: European Platform for Investing in Children (2015). 'France: significant support for women and high monetary benefits' (online). www.europa.eu/epic/countries/france/index_en.htm (Accessed: August 2015).

43 Lundberg, C. (2013) 'It's Amazing to Be a Working Mom in France— Unless You Want a Job', USA: Slate (online). 15 July 2013. www.slate.com/articles/double_x/doublex/2013/07/working_moms_in_france_the_government_benefits_are_great_job_prospects_not. html (Accessed: August 2015).

44 Chemin, A. (2015) 'France's baby boom secret: get women into work and ditch rigid family norms', *Guardian*, Saturday 21 March 2015. www.theguardian.com/world/2015/mar/21/france-population-europe-fertility-rate (Accessed: August 2015).

45 Agence-France Presse (2015) 'Japan suffers lowest number of births on record as population shrinks' (online). *Guardian*, Thursday 1 January 2015. www.theguardian.com/world/2015/jan/01/japan-suffers-lowest-number-of-births-on-record-as-population-shrinks (Accessed: August 2015).

46 AWOC.org Ageing Without Children (website) www.awoc.org (Accessed: August 2015).

47 O'Connor, J. (2012) 'Trend of couples not having children just plain selfish' (online). *National Post* (Canada): 19 September 2012. www.news.nationalpost.com/full-comment/joe-oconnor-selfishness-behind-growing-trend-for-couples-to-not-have-children (Accessed: August 2015).

48 Keizer, R. (2010) 'Remaining childless: Causes and consequences from a life course perspective': Dissertation: Utrecht University. Data is not within dissertation as it is an estimate only, and based on data drawn from the Netherlands and the United States, but is referred to here in an article about Professor Keizer's research. www.nwo.nl/actueel/nieuws/2010/Kinderloosheid+is+zelden+een+keuze.html.

49 Wikipedia (2013) 'Plato' (online). Available at: www.en.wikipedia.org/wiki/Plato (Accessed: October 2015).

50 Cusk, R. (2003) *A Life's Work: On Becoming a Mother.* UK: Picador.

51 Cusk, R. (2008) 'I was only being honest', *Guardian*, Friday 21 March 2008. www.guardian.co.uk/books/2008/mar/21/biography.women. (Accessed: October 2015).

52 Arnold, L. and Campbell C. (2013) 'The High Price of Being Single in America', *The Atlantic*. Monday 14 January 2013. www.theatlantic.com/sexes/archive/2013/01/the-high-price-of-being-single-in-america/267043/ (Accessed May 2013).

53 Kargmen, J. (2007) *Momzillas.* UK, London: Harper Perennial.

54 Carroll, L. (2012) *The Baby Matrix.* USA: LiveTrue Books. www.livetruebooks.com.

55 Kirchgaessnner, S. (2015) 'Pope Francis: not having children is selfish', *Guardian* (online). Wednesday 11 February 2015. www.theguardian.com/world/2015/feb/11/pope-francis-the-choice-to-not-have-children-is-selfish (Accessed: August 2015).

56 Lee, S. (2003) 'Myths and reality in male infertility' pp.73–85 in *Inconceivable Conceptions: Psychological Aspects of Infertility and Reproductive Technology.* Eds. Jane Haynes and Juliet Miller. Afterword by Germaine Greer. (2003) UK, Hove: Brunner-Routledge.

57 Salecl, R. (2010) *Choice.* UK, London: Profile Books.

58 Day, J. (2011) 'Light at the End of the Tunnel', Gateway Women, 5 April 2011 (online). www.gateway-women.com/light-at-the-end-of-the-tunnel/ (Accessed: October 2015).

59 See Tonkin, L (2014) 'Fantasy and Loss in Circumstantial Childlessness: A thesis submitted in fulfillment of the requirements for the Degree of Doctor of Philosophy in Sociology in the University of Canterbury (NZ)' for an excellent exploration as to how Doka's (1989, 2002) theory of 'disenfranchised grief' can be applied to childless women. Downloadable PDF at www.loistonkin.com/ (Accessed: August 2015).

60 Prechtel, M. (2015) *The Smell of Rain on Dust: Grief and Praise.* USA: North Atlantic Books. www.floweringmountain.com (Accessed: August 2015).

61 Wikipedia (2013) 'Pregnancy over age 50' (online). Available at: www.en.wikipedia.org/wiki/Pregnancy_over_age_50 (Accessed: October 2015).

62 UK: Harris, Sarah (no date) 'Third of women have an abortion by the age of 45', *Daily Mail* (online). www.dailymail.co.uk/news/article-82368/Third-women-abortion-age-45.html ; USA: Guttmacher Institute. 'Abortion in the United States' (online). www.guttmacher.org/media/presskits/abortion-US/statsandfacts.html (Accessed: August 2015).

63 Dawn, E. (2015) 'Pro-Voice, not Pro-Life vs. Pro-Choice: A Better Way to Talk About Abortion', UPLIFT, 12 August 2015 (online). www.upliftconnect.com/pro-voice/ (Accessed: August 2015).

64 Saying Goodbye (website) www.sayinggoodbye.org (Accessed: August 2015).

65 The Pursuit of Motherhood [Blog]. Jessica Hepburn: 'Joy and Melancholy', 6 July 2014. www.thepursuitofmotherhood.wordpress.com/2014/07/06/joy-and-melancholy/ (Accessed: August 2015).

66 The Bitter Babe [Blog] 2012–2014 www.thebitterbabe.com/ (Accessed: August 2015).

67 Eckel, S. (2014) *It's Not You: 27 (Wrong) Reasons You're Single.* USA, New York: Perigree (Penguin Group). www.saraeckel.com.

68 Hadley, R. (2015) Private email correspondence with author. Robin Hadley's website is: www.wantedtobeadad.com (Accessed: October 2015).

69 Rettner, R. NBC News Health (online). 'Fertility treatments may put women at risk for PTSD symptoms, study suggests', Wednesday 8 August 2012 www.vitals.nbcnews.com/_news/2012/08/08/13184349-fertility-treatments-may-put-women-at-risk-for-ptsd-symptoms-study-suggests?lite (Accessed: August 2015).

70 Berman, E. (2015) 'How Infertility Can Kill Your Sex Drive', *Huffington Post* (online). 9 June 2015. www.huffingtonpost.ca/erica-berman/infertility-trouble-conceiving_b_7544548.html (Accessed: August 2015).

71 Lieblum, S. R., Aviv, A., and Hameri, R. (1998) 'Life after infertility treatment: a long-term investigation of marital and sexual function', Human Reproduction, Vol. 13, No. 12, pp. 3569–3574, 1998. www.humrep.oxfordjournals.org/content/13/12/3569.full.pdf (Accessed: August 2015).

72 The Center for Complicated Grief (website) 'Are you asking yourself "what is complicated grief?"' (online). www.complicatedgrief.org/complicated-grief/ (Accessed: August 2015).

73 The Center for Complicated Grief (website) 'Prevalence and Risk' (online). www.complicatedgrief.org/complicated-grief/prevalence-and-risk/ (Accessed: August 2015).

74 Kübler-Ross, E. (1969) *On Death and Dying*. New York: Routledge.

75 Elisabeth Kübler-Ross Foundation (2013) 'Welcome' (online). Available at: www.ekrfoundation.org/ (Accessed: October 2015).

76 Sapsted, D., Foster, P. and Jones, G. (2011) 'Grief is price of love, says the Queen', *Telegraph*. Wednesday 21 September 2001. www.telegraph.co.uk/news/worldnews/northamerica/usa/1341155/Grief-is-price-of-love-says-the-Queen.html (Accessed: October 2015).

77 Beattie, M. (1990) *The Language of Letting Go*. USA, Minnesota: Hazelden Publishing.

78 Press Association (2015). 'Grief "is incredibly individual"', *Mail Online* (online). 11 July 2015. www.dailymail.co.uk/wires/pa/article-3157180/Grief-incredibly-individual.html (Accessed: August 2015).

79 Kani Comstock's book *Honouring Missed Motherhood* (2013) has a section on creating rituals, including the full text of an alternative 'Mother's Day Service: Honouring the Feminine' (p122). In the UK, Saying Goodbye organise non-denominational services of remembrance in cathedrals for baby losses of all kinds, and London-based counsellor Gill Tunstall offers regular nature-based services. In the US, Our Spirit Babies offers ceremonies in the San Francisco Bay area, including those losses due to abortion.

80 Kondo, M. (2014) *The Life-Changing Magic of Tidying: A simple, effective way to banish clutter forever*. UK: Vermillion.

81 Cleantis, T. (2015) *The Next Happy: Let Go of the Life You Planned and Find a New Way Forward*. USA, Minnesota: Hazelden Publishing.

82 Pinterest (website) Gateway Women: Grief & Loss (online). www.pinterest.com/gatewaywomen/gateway-women-grief-loss/ (Accessed: August 2015).

83 Malik, S. H., and Coulson, N. S. (2013) 'Coming to Terms with Permanent Involuntary Childlessness: A Phenomenological Analysis

of Bulletin Board Postings' (online). EJOP: Europe's Journal of Psychology. Vol. 9, No. 1 (2013) www.ejop.psychopen.eu/article/view/534/html (Accessed: October 2015).

84 Pet Partners (website) 'Benefits of the Human–Animal Bond' (online). www.petpartners.org/learn/benefits-human-animal-bond/ (Accessed: August 2015).

85 The Grief Club (website) www.melodybeattie.net/ (Accessed: August 2015).

86 Goodreads (website) 'Shannon L. Alder Quotes' (online). www.goodreads.com/quotes/1065997-don-t-waste-your-time-trying-to-explain-yourself-to-people (Accessed: August 2015).

87 Brown, B. (2012) 'Listening to Shame' [Online Video] www.ted.com/talks/brene_brown_listening_to_shame?language=en (Accessed: August 2015).

88 Linder, D. (2012) 'Famous Trials, Poems Written by Lord Alfred Douglas' (online). University of Missouri-Kansas City (UMKC) School of Law. Available at: www.law2.umkc.edu/faculty/projects/ftrials/wilde/poemsofdouglas.htm (Accessed: October 2015).

89 GOV.UK (website) 12 November 2014, 'Flexible Working' (online). www.gov.uk/flexible-working/overview (Accessed: August 2015).

90 Dunbar, P. (2013) 'Why SHOULD childless women like us do longer hours to cover for working mothers?' *Daily Mail* (online). 28 July 2013. www.dailymail.co.uk/femail/article-2380473/Why-SHOULD-childless-women-like-longer-hours-cover-working-mothers.html (Accessed: August 2015).

91 *Today* [Radio Programme] 'Women without children "resent" the flexibility given to colleagues that do', BBC Radio 4. Live broadcast 2 April 2014 (online). www.audioboom.com/boos/2039222-women-without-children-resent-the-flexibility-given-to-colleagues-that-do (Accessed: August 2015).

92 Shellenbarger, S. (2008) 'Janet Napolitano and the Persistence of "Singlism"' (online). *Wall Street Journal*. 5 December 2008. (Accessed: August 2015).

93 Oxford Dictionaries (online) 'spinster'. www.oxforddictionaries.com/definition/english/spinster (Accessed: October 2015).

94 Office for National Statistics (2013) 'An overview of 40 years of data

(General Lifestyle Survey Overview – a report on the 2011 General Lifestyle Survey)' (online). www.ons.gov.uk/ons/rel/ghs/general-lifestyle-survey/2011/rpt-40-years.html (Accessed: August 2015).

95 Trowbridge, A. (2013) CBS NEWS (USA), 'Living alone? You're not the only one' (online). 29 August 2013. www.cbsnews.com/news/living-alone-youre-not-the-only-one/ (Accessed: August 2015).

96 Gerstel, N. Professor of Sociology, University of Massachusetts (2011) 'Single And Unmarried Americans as Family and Community Members: A Fact Sheet Prepared for the Council on Contemporary Families in Honor of Unmarried and Singles Week, September 18–24', 15 September 2011. USA: Council on Contemporary Families, (online). www.contemporaryfamilies.org/single-unmarried-americans-family-community-members/ (Accessed: August 2015).

97 Parker-Pope, T. (2011) 'In a Married World, Singles Struggle for Attention', *New York Times* (online). 19 September 2011. www.well. blogs.nytimes.com/2011/09/19/the-plight-of-american-singles/ (Accessed: August 2015).

98 DePaulo, B. (2011) Bella DePaulo: Singles Research and Writing (website), 'On 'Singlism: What It Is, Why It Matters, and How to Stop It' (online). www.belladepaulo.com/singles-research-and-writing/ (Accessed: August 2015).

99 Wroe, N. (2012) 'Janet Baker: A life in music', *Guardian*, Friday 13 July 2012. www.guardian.co.uk/culture/2012/jul/13/janet-baker-life-in-writing (Accessed: October 2015).

100 Carroll, H. (2012) 'I may not be a mother - but I'm still a person ...', *Irish Independent* (online). Available at: www.independent.ie/lifestyle/parenting/i-may-not-be-a-mother-but-im-still-a-person-3041601.html (Accessed: October 2015).

101 Italie, L. (2015) 'New book on dating blames the numbers – not the women' (online). *AP Big Story: The Associated Press*, 25 August 2015. www.bigstory.ap.org/article/3b2d5f5fa78c4bf5851ee69c20122c cc/new-book-dating-blames-numbers-not-women (Accessed: October 2015).

102 Ryan, C. and Jethá, C. (2010) *Sex at Dawn: How We Mate, Why We Stray and What It Means for Modern Relationships.* USA, New York: HarperPerennial Edition, 2011.

103 Savvy Auntie (website) www.savvyauntie.com.

104 Hilliard, C. (2012) 'I'm Not a Lesbian, I'm Just Childless', *Huffington Post*, 20 July (online). Available at: www.huffingtonpost.com/Chlo%C3%A9%20Hilliard/not-lesbian-just-childless_b_1687646.html (Accessed: August 2015).

105 Green, R, J. (1996) 'How Many Witches' (online). Available at www.nizkor.org/ftp.cgi?miscellany/witches/how-many-witches (Accessed: October 2015).

106 Stavrakopoulou, F. (Forthcoming) *Baal and Asherah: Image, Sex, Power, and the Other*. UK, Oxford: Oxford University Press. More: www.humanities.exeter.ac.uk/theology/staff/stavrakopoulou (Accessed: October 2015).

107 Howard, S. (2012) 'Kids: Who Needs Them? We NoMos – Not Mothers – Are Out and We are Proud and We're Busy Making Our Own Friends and Support Networks', *Sunday Times Style Magazine*, Sunday 6 May 2012. Available at: www.mantramanga.files.wordpress.com/2011/04/kids-who-needs-them.jpg (Accessed: October 2015).

108 Day, J. (2012) 'The Gateway Women Manifesto: Are Childless Women the New Suffragettes?' Gateway Women, 3 May 2012 (online). Available at: www.gateway-women.com/the-nomos-manifesto-are-childless-women-the-new-suffragettes/ (Accessed: October 2015).

109 Frankl, V. (1946) *Man's Search for Meaning*. Translated from the German by I. Lasch. With a Preface by Gordon W. Allport and Preface to the 1992 Edition by V. Frankl (2004) UK, London: Ebury Publishing.

110 Wikipedia 'Combined oral contraceptive pill' (online). www.en.wikipedia.org/wiki/Combined_oral_contraceptive_pill (Accessed: October 2015).

111 Kipnis, L. (2015) 'Maternal Instincts' pp.31–46 in *Selfish, Shallow and Self Absorbed: Sixteen Writers on the Decision NOT to have Kids*. Ed. and Introduction, Meghan Daum. USA, New York: Picador.

112 Carroll, L. (2012) *The Baby Matrix: Why Freeing Our Minds from Outmoded Thinking About Parenthood & Reproduction Will Create a Better World*. USA: Live True Books. (p.24) Quoting Dr. Frederick Wyatt in Allan Carlson, Ph.D, 'Marriage and Procreation: On Children as the First Purpose of Marriage,' lecture given to the Family Research Council, Washington, DC, on 20 October 2004, adapted in 'The Family

in America', 18, no. 12 December 2004). www.lauracarroll.com/books/
bit.ly/babymatrix (Accessed: August 2015).

113 Carroll, L. (2012) *The Baby Matrix: Why Freeing Our Minds From Outmoded Thinking About Parenthood & Reproduction Will Create a Better World*. USA: Live True Books. (p.10) www.lauracarroll.com/ books, bit.ly/babymatrix (Accessed: August 2015).

114 Hollis, J. (2005) *Finding Meaning in the Second Half of Life: How to Finally, Really Grow Up*. USA, New York: Gotham Books (Penguin) p.17.

115 Dr Phil (2013) 'National Parenting Survey' (online). Available at: www.drphil.com/articles/article/311 (Accessed: October 2015).

116 Carroll, L. (2013) 'Getting Real About Regret' (online). Available at: www.lauracarroll.com/getting-real-about-regret/#sthash.5NsXwdS8. dpuf (Accessed: October 2015).

117 Dutton, I. (2013) 'The mother who says having these two children is the biggest regret of her life', *Daily Mail* (online). 3 April 2013. www.dailymail.co.uk/femail/article-2303588/The-mother-says-having-children-biggest-regret-life.html (Accessed: August 2015).

118 Hartley, J. (2015) 'When you regret having children', *The Age* (Australia), (online). 16 August 2015. www.theage.com.au/it-pro/i-regret-having-children-20150816-gjo208 (Accessed: August 2015).

119 Asher, R. (2011) *Shattered: Modern Motherhood and the Illusion of Equality*. UK, London: Random House Publishing Group.

120 Gateway Women (website) www.gateway-women.com (Accessed: October 2015).

121 Manterfield, L. (2010) *I'm Taking My Eggs and Going Home: How One Woman Dared to Say No to Motherhood*. USA: Steel Rose Press. www.lifewithoutbaby.com.

122 Brown, B. (2013) 'The Power of Vulnerability', Live talk at The RSA in London, UK. www.thersa.org/events/2013/07/the-power-of-vulnerability/ (Accessed: October 2015).

123 Day, J. (2014) 'The Childless Menopause', Gateway Women (online). 8 September 2014. www.gateway-women.com/the-childless-menopause/ (Accessed: October 2015).

124 de Chardin, P. T. (1955) *The Phenomenon of Man*. UK, London (1959): William Collins. www.en.wikipedia.org/wiki/The_Phenomenon_of_ Man (Accessed: October 2015).

125 Cameron, J. (1995) *The Artist's Way: A Course in Discovering and Recovering Your Creative Self.* UK, London: Pan Books.

126 Neff, K. (2011) *Self-Compassion: stop beating yourself up and leave insecurity behind.* UK: Hodder and Stoughton.

127 Brown, B. (2010) *The Gifts of Imperfection: Let Go of Who You Think You're Supposed to Be and Embrace Who You Are.* USA, Minnesota: Hazelden Publishing.

128 Dickson, M. (2010) *Please Take One: Step Towards a More Generous Life.* UK, London: The Generous Press. www.pleasetakeonestep.com/ (Accessed: October 2015).

129 Roth, G. (2011) *Women, Food and God: An Unexpected Path to Almost Everything.* USA, New York: Simon & Schuster.

130 Beck, M. (2011) *Finding Your Way in a Wild New World: Reclaim Your True Nature to Create the Life You Want.* USA, New York: Simon & Schuster. bit.ly/wordlessness. www.marthabeck.com (Accessed: October 2015).

131 Neff, K. (2011) *Self-Compassion: stop beating yourself up and leave insecurity behind.* UK: Hodder and Stoughton. pp.47–49.

132 Gottman, J. (1994) *Why Marriages Succeed Or Fail and How to Make Yours Last.* USA, New York: Simon & Schuster.

133 Fredrickson, B. (2009) *Positivity: Groundbreaking Research Reveals How to Embrace the Hidden Strength of Positive Emotions, Overcome Negativity, and Thrive.* USA: Crown Publishing Group.

134 Neff, K. (2011) *Self-Compassion: stop beating yourself up and leave insecurity behind.* UK: Hodder and Stoughton, pp.50–51.

135 Wikipedia 'Donald Winnicott' (online). Available at: www.en.wikipedia. org/wiki/Donald_Winnicott (Accessed: October 2015).

136 Ban Breathnach, S. (2003) *Romancing the Ordinary: A Year of Everyday Indulgences.* USA, New York: Simon & Schuster.

137 The Artist's Way (online video) 'Morning Pages'. www.juliacameronlive.com/basic-tools/morning-pages/ (Accessed: October 2015).

138 MacLeod, H. (2009) *Ignore everybody: and 39 other keys to creativity.* USA, New York: Portfolio (Penguin Books).

139 The Artist's Way (online video) 'Morning Pages' www.juliacameronlive.com/basic-tools/morning-pages/ (Accessed: October 2015).

140 Wikipedia 'Cyril Connolly' (online). Available at: www.en.wikipedia.org/wiki/Cyril_Connolly (Accessed: October 2015).

141 Woolf, V. (1942) *Professions for Women*. Collected in *Women in Writing* (2003) Ed. Michele Barrett. UK: Houghton Mifflin Harcourt.

142 Pinterest (website). 'Gateway Women: Childless and Childfree Women Role Models' (online). www.pinterest.com/gatewaywomen/gateway-women-childless-childfree-women-role-model/ (Accessed: August 2015).

143 Carson, R. (1962) *Silent Spring*. USA, New York: Houghton Mifflin Company.

144 Brown, S. (2008) 'Play is more than fun' (online video). Available at: www.ted.com/talks/stuart_brown_says_play_is_more_than_fun_it_s_vital.html (Accessed: October 2015).

145 Ehrenreich, B. (2010) *Smile or Die: How Positive Thinking Fooled America and the World*. UK: Granta Books.

146 MacLeod, H. (2009) *Ignore everybody: and 39 other keys to creativity*. USA, New York: Portfolio (Penguin Books).

147 Pinterest (website). 'Gateway Women: Childless and Childfree Women Role Models' (online). www.pinterest.com/gatewaywomen/gateway-women-childless-childfree-women-role-model/ (Accessed: August 2015).

148 Dyer, G. (2012) *Out of Sheer Rage: In the Shadow of D.H. Lawrence*. UK: Canongate Books.

149 Wikipedia 'Joseph Campbell' (online). Available at: www.en.wikipedia.org/wiki/Joseph_Campbell (Accessed: October 2015).

150 Moyers, J. C. (1989) *Joseph Campbell: Follow Your Bliss Conversations With Bill Moyers*. USA: Harper Collins.

151 Adams, D. (2007) *The Hitchhiker's Guide to the Galaxy*. UK, London: Random House Publishing Group. See also www.independent.co.uk/life-style/history/42-the-answer-to-life-the-universe-and-everything-2205734.html (Accessed: August 2015).

152 Wikipedia 'Maslow's hierarchy of needs' (online). Available at: www.en.wikipedia.org/wiki/Maslow%27s_hierarchy_of_needs (Accessed: October 2015).

153 Robbins, T. (2006) 'Why We Do What We Do' (online video). Available at: bit.ly/tony-ted (Accessed: November 2015).

154 www.nonviolentcommunication.com/aboutnvc/feelings_needs.htm (Accessed: October 2015).

155 Wikipedia 'George E. P. Box' (online). Available at: www.en.wikipedia. org/wiki/George_E._P._Box (Accessed: October 2015).

156 Pressfield, S. (2003) *The War of Art: Winning the Inner Creative Battle*. USA: Orion.

157 Chocano, C. (2012) 'Girls Love Math. We Never Stop Doing It', *New York Times*, November 16 (online). Available at: www.nytimes. com/2012/11/18/magazine/girls-love-math-we-never-stop-doing-it. html?pagewanted=all&_r=2& (Accessed: September 2015).

158 Steinem, G. (1971) 'Sisterhood', *New York Magazine*, 20 December 1971, p. 49. www.en.wikipedia.org/wiki/Gloria_Steinem (Accessed: October 2015).

159 Karpf, A. (2014) *How to Age*. UK, London: The School of Life, Pan Macmillan. p.105.

160 AWOC: Ageing Without Children (website) www.awoc.org (Accessed: August 2015).

161 www.awoc.org/statistics (Accessed: October 2015).

162 Brunel University London 'Mary Pat Sullivan: Programme Leader MA Social Work' (online). www.brunel.ac.uk/people/mary-pat-sullivan (Accessed: October 2015).

163 AWOC: Ageing Without Children (website) www.awoc.org (Accessed: August 2015).

164 Ipsos Mori (website) Family estrangement survey for Stand Alone, 7 October 2014, (online). www.ipsos-mori.com/researchpublications/ researcharchive/3456/Family-estrangement-survey-for-Stand-Alone. aspx (Accessed: August 2015).

165 Stand Alone (website) www.standalone.org.uk/ (Accessed: August 2015).

166 *ITV News* [TV programme] 'One in five families affected by "estrangement"', 7 October 2014, (online). www.itv.com/news/tyne-tees/2014-10-07/one-in-five-families-affected-by-estrangement/ (Accessed: August 2015).

167 Bingham, J. (2012) 'British grandparents shouldering childcare burden' (online). *Telegraph* (28 June 2012) www.telegraph.co.uk/women/mother-tongue/9360347/British-grandparents-shouldering-childcare-burden. html.

168 AWOC: Ageing Without Children (website) www.awoc.org (Accessed: August 2015).

169 *BBC News* [TV programme] 'The dangers of loneliness as a parent', 25 August 2015, (online). www.bbc.com/news/uk-34049033 (Accessed: August 2015).

170 Campaign to End Loneliness (website) 'About loneliness' (online) www.campaigntoendloneliness.org/about-loneliness/ (Accessed: October 2015).

171 Karpf, A. (2014) *How to Age*. UK, London: The School of Life, Pan Macmillan. p.139.

172 Older Women's CoHousing (website) www.owch.org.uk/ (Accessed: August 2015).

173 UK Cohousing Network (website) www.cohousing.org.uk/ (Accessed: August 2015).

174 Hardy, R. (2014) 'Shared lives: community-based approach to supporting adults', *Guardian*, Friday 23 May 2014 (online). www.theguardian.com/social-care-network/2014/may/23/shared-lives-community-based-supporting-adults (Accessed: August 2015).

175 *ABC News* [TV programme] 'Seattle Pre-School in a Nursing Home "Transforms" Residents', 16 June 2015. www.abcnews.go.com/Lifestyle/seattle-preschool-nursing-home-transforms-elderly-residents/story?id=31803817 (Accessed: August 2015).

176 Daum, M. (2015) *Selfish, Shallow and Self Absorbed: Sixteen Writers on the Decision NOT to have Kids*. Ed. and Introduction, Meghan Daum. USA, New York: Picador.

177 Day, J. (2012) 'Julia Gillard and the fear of the childless woman' (online). *Guardian*, 25 October 2012. www.theguardian.com/commentisfree/2012/oct/25/julia-gillard-childless-woman (Accessed: October 2015).

178 Pinterest (website) 'Gateway Women Childless and Childfree Role Models' (online). Available at: www.pinterest.com/gatewaywomen/gateway-women-childless-childfree-women-role-model/ (Accessed: August 2015).

179 Eshure – European Society of Human Reproduction and Embryology (2014) 'Art Fact Sheet' (online). Available at: www.eshre.eu/sitecore/content/Home/Guidelines%20and%20Legal/ART%20fact%20sheet (Accessed: October 2015).

180 Resolve: The National Infertility Association (website) 'Male Factor' (online) www.resolve.org/about-infertility/medical-conditions/male-factor.html (October: 2015).

181 Macy, J. and Johnstone, C. (2012) *Active Hope: How to Face the Mess We're In Without Going Crazy.* USA, California: New World Library, p.14.

182 Wilber, K. (1995) *Sex, Ecology, Spirituality: The Spirit of Evolution.* USA, Boston: Shambhala Publications. Second Edition, Revised (2000).